Concise Review of Physiology

Manjeet Kaur, MD

PEEPEE
PUBLISHERS AND DISTRIBUTORS (P) LTD.

Concise Review of Physiology

Published by
Pawaninder P. Vij & Anupam Vij

Peepee Publishers and Distributors (P) Ltd.
Head Office: 160, Shakti Vihar, Pitam Pura
Delhi - 110 034 (India)

Correspondence Address:
7/31, First Floor, Ansari Road, Daryaganj,
New Delhi-110 002 (India)
Ph: 41512412, 9811156083
e-mail: peepee160@yahoo.co.in
e-mail: peepee160@gmail.com
www.peepeepub.com

First Edition: **2019**

ISBN: 9788184452501

PREFACE

The aim of this book is to provide multiple choice questions on all aspects of human/medical physiology. I hope that the questions will be useful for undergraduates in medical, dental, nursing and science courses in human/medical physiology and also to the postgraduate students preparing for Indian and international entrance examinations.

Questions are grouped in 39 chapters and each chapter provides the basic and applied aspects of physiology. The reasoning/explanation of answers are carefully given. For further reference and clarification refer **Ganong and Guyton.** However, comments and suggestions from the colleagues and students will be helpful to update the knowledge in the future print of the book.

Dr. Manjeet Kaur

DEDICATED TO

I would like to thank my parents, teachers, friend and God Almighty who have been always there for me. And my **students** who have always been my inspiration to start and pursue my little journey towards this book.

Dr. Manjeet Kaur

CONTENTS

UNIT I. INTRODUCTION

Chapter 1 : The General and Cellular Basis of Medical Physiology 1

UNIT II. PHYSIOLOGY OF NERVE AND MUSCLE CELLS

Chapter 2 : Excitable Tissue: Nerve 11

Chapter 3 : Excitable Tissue: Muscle 16

Chapter 4 : Synaptic and Junctional Transmission 22

Chapter 5 : Initiation of Impulses in Sense Organs 29

UNIT III. NERVOUS SYSTEM

Chapter 6 : Reflexes 34

Chapter 7 : Cutaneous, Deep and Visceral Sensation 38

Chapter 8 : Vision 44

Chapter 9 : Hearing and Equilibrium 50

Chapter 10 : Smell and Taste 58

Chapter 11 : Alert Behavior, Sleep and the Electrical Activity of the Brain 63

Chapter 12 : Control of Posture and Movement 68

Chapter 13 : The Autonomic Nervous System 73

Chapter 14 : Central Regulation of Visceral Function 79

Chapter 15 : Neural Basis of Instinctual Behavior and Emotions 83

Chapter 16 : Higher Functions of the Nervous System 90

UNIT IV. ENDOCRINOLOGY, METABOLISM AND REPRODUCTIVE FUNCTION

Chapter 17 : Energy Balance, Metabolism and Nutrition 97

Chapter 18 : The Thyroid Gland 104

Chapter 19 : Endocrine Functions of the Pancreas and the Regulation of Carbohydrate Metabolism 114

Chapter 20 : The Adrenal Medulla and Adrenal Cortex 121

Chapter 21 : Hormonal Control of Calcium Metabolism and the Physiology of Bone 129

Chapter 22 : Pituitary Gland 137

Chapter 23 : The Gonads: Development and Function of the Reproductive System 143

Chapter 24 : Endocrine Functions of the Kidneys, Heart and Pineal Gland 155

UNIT V. GASTROINTESTINAL FUNCTION

Chapter 25 : Digestion and Absorption 162

Chapter 26 : Regulation of Gastrointestinal Function 167

UNIT VI. CIRCULATION

Chapter 27 : Circulating Body Fluids 174

Chapter 28 : Origin of the Heartbeat and the Electrical Activity of the Heart 183

Chapter 29 : The Heart as a Pump 193

Chapter 30 : Dynamics of Blood and Lymph Flow 199

Chapter 31 : Cardiovascular Regulatory Mechanisms 208

Chapter 32 : Circulation Through Special Regions 215

Chapter 33 : Cardiovascular Homeostasis in Health and Disease 226

UNIT VII. RESPIRATION

Chapter 34 : Pulmonary Function 234

Chapter 35 : Gas Transport Between the Lungs and the Tissues 243

Chapter 36 : Regulation of Respiration 247

Chapter 37 : Respiratory Adjustments in Health and Disease 255

UNIT VIII. FORMATION AND EXCRETION OF URINE

Chapter 38 : Renal Function and Micturition 263

Chapter 39 : Regulation of Extracellular Fluid Composition and Volume 275

UNIT I. INTRODUCTION

Chapter 1 The General and Cellular Basis of Medical Physiology

1. **Cell membranes:**

   A. Contain relatively few protein molecules
   B. Contain many carbohydrate molecules
   C. Are freely permeable to electrolytes but not to proteins
   D. In some tissues permit the transport of glucose at a greater rate in the presence of insulin
   E. Have a stable composition throughout the life of the cell

Ans. (D)

Explanation:

Cell membranes are made up of lipids and proteins and is semipermeable, allowing some substances to pass through it and excluding others. The amount of protein varies with the function of the membrane but makes up on overage 50% of the mass of the membrane. Membranes are **dynamic** structures and their constituents are being constantly renewed at different rates. Some proteins are anchored to the cytoskeleton, but others move laterally in the membrane, e.g., receptors move in the membrane and aggregate at sites of endocytosis. *(Pg. 8-10)*

2. **The primary force moving water molecules from the blood plasma to the interstitial fluid is:**

   A. Active transport
   B. Cotransport with H^+
   C. Facilitated diffusion
   D. Cotransport with Na^+
   E. Filtration

Ans. (E)

Explanation:

The capillary wall separating plasma from interstitial fluid is different from the cell membranes separating interstitial fluid from intracellular fluid because the pressure difference across it makes **filtration** a significant factor in promoting movement of H_2O and solute.

(Pg. 35)

3. **Second messengers:**

A. Are substances that interact with first messengers outside cells

B. Are substances that bind to first messengers in the cell membrane

C. Are hormones secreted by cells in response to stimulation by another hormone

D. Mediate the intracellular responses to many different hormones and neurotransmitters

E. Are not formed in the brain

Ans. (D)

Explanation:

Many ligands in ECF bind to receptors on the surface of cells and many of them trigger the release of intracellular mediators such as cAMP, IP_3 and DAG that initiate changes in cell functions Consequently, the extracellular ligands are called **"first messengers"** and the intracellular mediators are called **"second messengers"**.

(Pg. 37)

4. **Which of the following is most directly involved in the regulation of apoptosis?**

A. Glucose-6-phosphatase

B. Adenylyl cyclase

C. Nitric oxide synthase

D. Aquaporin 2

E. Cytochrome c

Ans. (E)

Explanation:

Cells can die and be absorbed under genetic control. This process is called **programmed cell death** or **"Apoptosis".**

- It can be called **"cell suicide"** in the sense that the cell's own genes play an active role in its demise.
- **Apoptosis** is a very common process during development and in adulthood, e.g., in CNS, large no. of neurons are produced and then die during the remodeling that occurs during development and synapse formation.
- The final common pathway bringing about apoptosis is activation of **caspases (by cytochrome c which causes activation of caspases)** a group of cysteine proteases.
- **Net result**

  –DNA fragmentation.

  –Cytoplasmic and chromatin condensation

  ↓

  Bleb formation→ cell breakdown

  ↓

  Removal of debris by phagocytes

Trigger for Apoptosis

- **Fas** (projects from natural killer cells and T-cells).
- **TNF.**

(Pg. 25)

5. Proteins that are secreted by cells are:

A. Not synthesized on membrane-bound ribosomes
B. Initially synthesized with a signal peptide or leader sequence at their C terminal
C. Found in vesicles and secretory granules
D. Moved across the cell membranes by endocytosis

E. Secreted in a form that is larger than the form present in the endoplasmic reticulum

Ans. (C)

Explanation:

Many and perhaps all proteins that are secreted by cells are synthesized as larger proteins and polypeptide sequences are cleared off from them during maturation. In case of hormones, these larger forms are called preprohormones and prohormones. Most secreted polypeptides and proteins have a leader sequence that targets them to the endoplasmic reticulum and are secreted by **exocytosis.**

(Pg. 25)

6. Which of the following cell membrane channels is a tetramer with a channel in each of the four subunits?

A. CLC Cl^- channels
B. Aquaporins
C. Potassium channels
D. Glucose transporters
E. $GABA_A$ channels

Ans. (B)

Explanation:

In many situations in the body, movement of water by simple diffusion is augmented by movement through water channels. They are now called **aquaporins** and five have been identified.

Aquaporin 1, 2, 3	:	found in kidneys
Aquaporin 4	:	found in brain
Aquaporin 5	:	found in salivary and lacrimal glands and in respiratory tract.

Vasopressin sensitive water channel in collecting tubule (kidneys) is **aquaporin-2.**

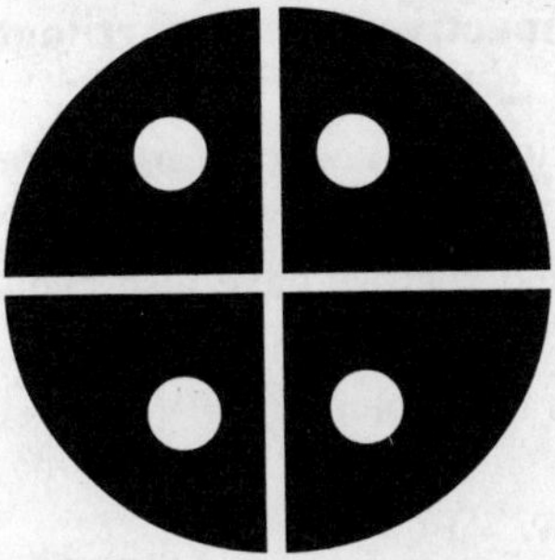

Structure of Aquaporin

Aquaporin water channels are tetramers with an intracellular channel in each submit.

(Pg. 32)

7. **Deuterium oxide and inulin are injected into a normal 30-year-old man. The volume of distribution of deuterium oxide is found to be 42 L and that of inulin 14 L.**

   A. The man's intracellular fluid volume is about 14 L

   B. The man's intracellular fluid is about 28 L

   C. The man's plasma volume is about 7 L

   D. The man's interstitial fluid volume is about 9 L

   E. The man's total body water cannot be determined from these data

Ans. **(B)**

Explanation:

- Extracellular fluid volume (ECF) is difficult to measure because the limits of this space are ill-defined and because few substances mix rapidly in all parts of the space while remaining exclusively extra-cellular. Many substances enter CSF slowly because of the blood-brain barrier. Equilibrium is slow with joint fluid and aqueous humor and with the ECF in relatively avascular tissues such as

dense connective tissue, cartilage and some parts of bone.

- **Perhaps the most accurate measurement of ECF is obtained by using inulin.**
- Mannitol and sucrose have also been used to measure ECF volume.
- Intracellular fluid volume (ICFV) is calculated by using
  ICFV= TBW –.ECF.
- TBW (Total body water) is measured using **Deuterium oxide** (D_2O, heavy water), **Tritium oxide** and **aminopyrine** have also been used for this purpose.
  Therefore ICFV= 42–14= 28 L.

8. Which of the following diseases is due to a mutation in the mitochondrial genome?

A. Cystic fibrosis
B. Leber's hereditary optic neuropathy
C. Hypothalamic diabetes insipidus
D. Familial male precocious puberty
E. Hirschsprung's disease

Ans. (B)

Explanation:

Leber's hereditary optic neuropathy is due to mutation in the mitochondrial genome. (*Parson's Book of Diseases of Eyes, 20th Ed/Pg. 348)*

Cystic Fibrosis: Most secreted polypeptides and proteins have a leader response that targets them to the endoplasmic reticulum and are secreted by exocytosis, a growing list of proteins that are secreted lack a signal sequence. In them secretion probably occurs via ATP-dependent membrane transporters. There is a large family of these ATP-binding cassette (ABC) transport proteins and they transport ions and other substances as well as proteins between organelles and across cell membranes. The cystic fibrosis transmembrane conductance regulator (CFTR) is one of those ABC transport proteins and in abnormal patients with cystic fibrosis.

9. Which of the following receptors does not span the cell membrane seven times?

A. β-adrenergic receptor
B. Rhodopsin
C. 5-HT_{IC} receptor
D. Mineralocorticoid receptor
E. LH receptor

Ans. (D)

Explanation:

Following are all serpentine receptors i.e. proteins that span the cell membrane seven times and are all coupled to heterotrimeric G proteins.

- β-adrenergic receptor
- Rhodopsin receptor
- Histamine receptor
- LH receptor

(Pg. 42)

10. Which of the following has both plasma membrane and intracellular receptors?

A. IL-1β
B. Growth hormone
C. Ghrelin
D. Dopamine
E. Estradiol

Ans. (E)

Explanation:

Most of the effects of **estrogens** are genomic i.e. due to actions on the nucleus, but some are so rapid that it is difficult to believe they are mediated via production of mRNA. Now evidence is there that these effects are mediated by cell membrane receptors that appear to be structurally related to the nuclear receptors and produce their effects by intracellular mitogen-activated protein kinase pathways.

(Pg. 442)

- **Growth hormone** activates JAK2-STAT pathway, which is a member of the Janus family. of cytoplasmic tyrosine kinases.
- **Ghrelin** is one of the endogenous ligands for the GH secretogogue receptors in the anterior pituitary gland. Operates like leptin as a peripherally generated regulator of appetite.

(Pg. 239)

- **Dopamine** acts via D_2 receptors. Five different dopamine receptors have been cloned. This provides for variety in the type of responses produced by dopamine. Most but perhaps not all of the responses to these receptors are mediated by heterotrimeric G proteins. Cytokines also activates JAK (Janus tyrosine Kinases) in the cytoplasm.

(Pg. 46)

11. Which of the following is a lysosomal storage disease?

A. Cystic fibrosis
B. Tay-Sachs disease
C. Duchenne's muscular dystrophy
D. Testotoxicosis
E. Long QT syndrome

Ans. (B)

Explanation:

When a lysosomal enzyme is congenitally absent, the lysosomes become engorged with the material the enzyme normally degrades. This eventually leads to one of the lysosomal storage diseases e.g. Tay-Sachs disease, which causes mental retardation and blindness.

12. Hydrogen ion concentration in lysosomes is:

A. Greater than H^+ ion concentration in cytoplasm of cells
B. Samé as H^+ ion concentration in cytoplasm of cells
C. Less than H^+ ion concentration in cytoplasm of cells

Ans. (A)

13. Contribution of normal concentration of plasma glucose to total plasma osmolality is:

A. Greater than contribution of normal concentration of plasma Na^+ to total plasma osmolality

B. Same as contribution of normal concentration of plasma Na^+ to total plasma osmolality

C. Less than contribution of normal concentration of plasma Na^+ to total plasma osmolality

Ans. (C)

Explanation:

Osmolality is the number of osmoles/kg of solvent so more osmotically active substances have more contribution to osmolality.

(Pg. 5)

14. Calculated plasma volume when some of the dye used to measure it is unknowingly injected subcutaneously instead of intravenously:

A. Greater than calculated plasma volume when all of the dye used to measure it is injected intravenously

B. Same as calculated plasma volume when all of the dye used to measure it is injected intravenously

C. Less than calculated plasma volume when all of the dye used to measure it is injected intravenously

Ans. (A)

15. Concentration of Ca^{2+} in intracellular fluid is:

A. Greater than concentration of Ca^{2+} in interstitial fluid

B. Same as concentration of Ca^{2+} in interstitial fluid

C. Less than concentration of Ca^{2+} in interstitial fluid

Ans. (C)

Explanation:

The free Ca^{2+} concentration in cytoplasm at rest is maintained at about 100 nmol/l.

The Ca^{2+} concentration in intracellular fluid is about 12,000 times the cytoplasmic concentration, so there is marked inwardly directed concentration gradient as well as inwardly directed electrical gradient. Much of the intracellular Ca^{2+} is bound by endoplasmic reticulum and other organelles and provide a store from which Ca^{2+} can be mobilized via ligand gated channels to increase concentration of free Ca^{2+} in cytoplasm. Increased cytoplasmic Ca^{2+} binds to and activates calcium binding proteins, and these in turn activates a number of protein kinases.

(Pg. 40)

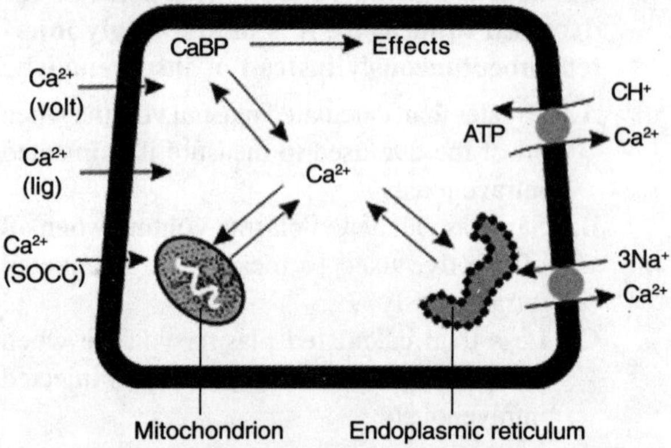

Ca^{2+} handling in mammalian cells

16. Size of mitochondrial genome is:

A. Greater than size of nuclear genome
B. Same as size of nuclear genome.
C. Less than size of nuclear genome

Ans. (C)

Chapter 2 Excitable Tissue: Nerve

1. **An axon is placed on stimulating electrodes and an intracellular electrode is inserted and connected through cathode-ray oscilloscope (CRO) to an indifferent electrode. When an axon is stimulated, the LP (latent period) is 1.5 ms. The intracellular electrode is 6 cm from anode of stimulator and 4.5 cm from cathode of stimulator. What is conduction velocity of the axon?**

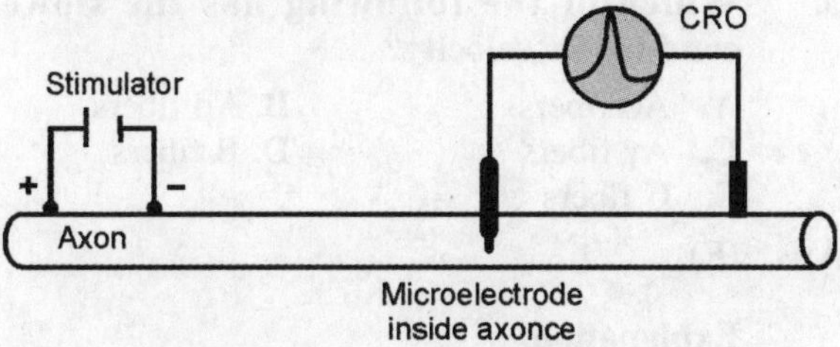

A. 15 m/s
B. 30 m/s
C. 40 m/s
D. 67.5 m/s
E. Cannot be determined

Ans. (B)

Explanation:

If duration of LP and distance between electrodes are known, the speed of conduction in the axon can be calculated. Cathode is normally the stimulating electrode because cathodal stimuli are depolarizing.
(Distance between cathodal stimulating electrode and exterior electrode is important).

Conduction velocity of ve axon $= \frac{4.5\text{cm-}30\text{m/s}}{1.5\text{ms}}$

2. **What percentage of the human genes are involved in the formation and function of the nervous system?**

A. 5 B. 15
C. 25 D. 40
E. 60

Ans. (D)

Explanation:

Human nervous system is a complex organ, it has been calculated that 40% of the human genes participate at least to a degree, in its formation.

(Pg. 51)

3. **Which of the following has the slowest conduction velocity?**

A. Aα fibers B. Aβ fibers
C. Aγ fibers D. B fibers
E. C fibers

Ans. (E)

Explanation:

C fibers are unmyelinated fibers while A and B are myelinated fibers.

4. **A man falls into a deep sleep with one arm under his head. This arm is paralyzed when he awakens, but it tingles, and pain sensation in it is still intact. The reason for the loss of motor function without loss of pain sensation is that in the nerves to his arm:**

A. A fibers are more susceptible to hypoxia than B fibers
B. A fibers are more sensitive to pressure than C fibers
C. C fibers are more sensitive to pressure than A fibers
D. Motor nerves are more affected by sleep than sensory nerves
E. Sensory nerves are nearer the bone than motor nerves and hence are less affected by pressure

Ans. (B)

5. **Which part of a neuron has the highest concentration of Na^+ channels per square millimeter of cell membrane?**

   A. Initial segment
   B. Dendrites
   C. Cell body near dendrites
   D. Axonal membrane under myelin
   E. None of the above

Ans. (A)

Explanation:

Voltage gated Na^+ channels are highly concentrated in the nodes of Ranvier and the initial segment in myelinated neurons. The no. of Na^+ channels/μm^2 are 350-500 in initial segment, 2000-12000 at nodes of Ranvier and 20-75 at axon terminals in myelinated mammalian neurons. Along the axons of unmyelinated neurons, the number is 110.

(Pg. 60)

6. **Which of the following statements about nerve growth factor is not true?**

   A. It is made up of three polypeptide subunits
   B. It is found of high concentration in the submandibular salivary glands of female mice
   C. It is necessary for the growth and development of the sympathetic nervous system
   D. It is picked up by nerves from the organs they innervate
   E. It is present in the brain

Ans. (B)

Explanation:

NGF (nerve growth factor) is made up of two α, two β and two γ subunits. In male mice, there is particularly high concentration in submandibular salivary glands and level is reduced by castration to that seen in females.

NGF is picked up by neurons in extracerebral organs they innervate and is transported in retrograde fashion from the endings of neurons to their cell bodies.

(Pg. 62-63)

7. **Number of glial cells in brain is:**

A. Greater than number of neurons in brain

B. Same as number of neurons in brain

C. Less than number of neurons in brain

Ans. (A)

Explanation:

CNS contains 10^{11} (100 billion) neurons. It also contains 10-15 times this number of glial cells.

(Pg. 63)

8. **Rate of conduction in small diameter axons is:**

A. Greater than the rate of conduction in large diameter axons

B. Same as the rate of conduction in large diameter axons

C. Less than the rate of conduction in large diameter axons

Ans. (C)

Explanation:

Mylinated axons conduct upto 50 times faster than the fastest unmylinated fibers.

9. **Excitability of neuron when resting membrane potential (RMP) is increased to –80 mV:**

A. Greater than excitability of neuron when RMP is reduced to – 60 mV

B. Same as excitability of neuron when RMP is reduced to – 60 mV

C. Less than excitability of neuron when RMP is reduced to – 60 mV

Ans. (C)

Explanation:

Excitability is inversely related to the threshold stimulus.

10. The total duration of compound action potential (AP) of a mixed nerve 5 mm from stimulating electrode:

A. Is greater than total duration of compound AP of mixed nerve 50 mm from stimulating electrode

B. Is same as total duration of compound AP of mixed nerve 50 mm from stimulating electrode

C. Is less than total duration of compound AP of mixed nerve 50 mm from stimulating electrode

Ans. (C)

Explanation:

If the distance between the stimulating and recording electrode is 5mm, the conduction velocity is V_1. Suppose the time interval between the stimulus and the appearance of the peaks is t_1.

$$\text{Therefore } t_1 = \frac{5\text{mm}}{V_1}$$

If the distance between the stimulating and recording electrode is 50 mm, the conduction velocity is V_2 (different since depends on distance) suppose the time interval between the stimulus and the appearance of the peaks is t_2.

$$\text{Therefore } t_2 = \frac{50\text{mm}}{V_2}$$

So t_2 is more than t_1.

UNIT II. PHYSIOLOGY OF NERVE AND MUSCLE CELLS

Chapter 3 Excitable Tissue: Muscle

1. The action potential of skeletal muscle:

A. Has a prolonged plateau phase

B. Spreads inward to all parts of the muscle via the T tubules

C. Causes the immediate uptake of Ca^{2+} into the lateral sacs of the sarcoplasmic reticulum

D. Is longer than the action potential of cardiac muscle

E. Is not essential for contraction

Ans. **(B)**

Explanation:

1. The process by which depolarization of the muscle initiates contraction is called as E-C coupling (excitation-contraction coupling). The AP (Action Potential) is transmitted to all the fibrils in the fiber *via* T system. It triggers the release of Ca^{+2} from the terminal cisterns the the lateral sacs of SR (Sarcoplasmic reticulum) next to theT system. Ca^{+2} initiates contraction by binding to troponin C. Shortly after releasing Ca^{+2}, the SR begins to reaccumulate it by ATP mediated active transport of it into the longitudnal portions of reticulum.
2. Prolonged pleatue which is the characterstic of cardiac muscle, is due to slower but prolonged opening of voltage-gated Ca^{+2} channels.

(Pg. 68)

3. AP of skeletal muscles lasts 2-4 ms, while in mammalians hearts, depolarization lasts 200 ms or more.

2. The functions of tropomyosin in skeletal muscle include:

A. Sliding on actin to produce shortening

B. Releasing C^{+2} after initiation of contraction
C. Binding to myosin during contraction
D. Acting as a "relaxing protein" at rest by covering up the sites where myosin binds to actin
E. Generating ATP, which it passes to the contractile mechanism

Ans. **(D)**

Explanation:

In resting muscle, troponin I is tightly bound to actin and tropomyosin covers the sits where myosin heads bind to actin. Thus the troponin-tropomyosin complex constitutes "relaxing protein" that inhibits the interaction between actin and myosin. When the Ca^{+2} released by AP binds to troponin C the binding of troponin I to actin is presumably weakened and this permits the tropomyosin to move laterally. This movement uncovers binding sits for myosin heads. ATP is then split and contraction occurs.

(Pg. 69)

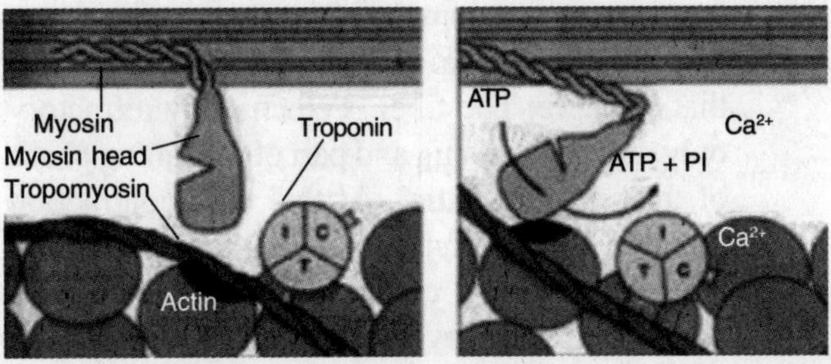

3. The cross-bridges of the sarcomere in skeletal muscle are made up of:

A. Actin
B. Myosin
C. Troponin
D. Tropomyosin
E. Myelin

Ans. **(B)**

4. The contractile response in skeletal muscle:

A. Starts after the action potential is over
B. Does not last as long as the action potential
C. Produces more tension when the muscles contracts isometrically than when the muscle contracts isotonically
D. Produces more work when the muscle contracts isometrically than when the muscle contracts isotonically
E. Decreases in magnitude with repeated stimulation

Ans. (C)

Explanation:

The action potential (AP) transmitted along the muscle fiber initiates contractile response.

(Pg. 68)

A single AP causes a brief contraction followed by relaxation. This response is called a **muscle twitch**. The twitch starts about 2 ms after the start of depolarization of the membrane, before repolarization is complete.The electrical response of a muscle fiber to repeated stimulation is like that of nerve. The fiber is electrically refractory only during the rising and part of the falling phase of the spike potential. At this time contraction initiated by the first stimulus is just beginning. However because contractile mechanism does not have a refractory period, repeated stimulation before relaxation has occurred, produces additional activation of contractile elements and a response that is added to the contraction already present. This phenomenon is known as **summation of contractions**.The tension developed during summation is considerably greater than that during single muscle twitch.

Muscle contraction involves shortening of contractile elements but muscles have elastic and viscous elements in series which the contracting

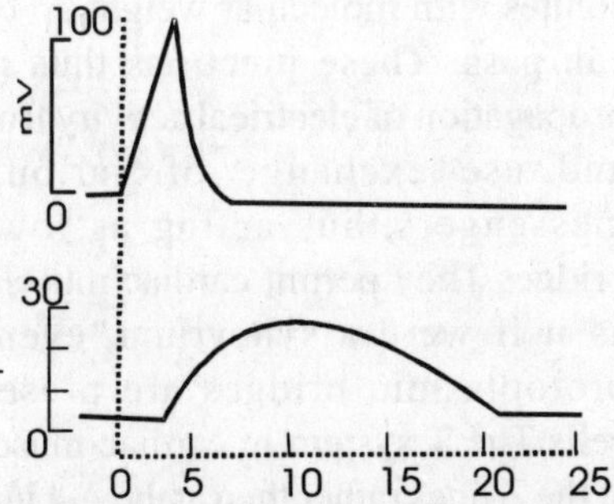

The electrical and mechanical responses of a mammalian skeletal muscle fiber to a single maximal stimulus. The electrical response (mV potential change) and the machanical response (T, tension in arbitrary unit) are plotted on the same abscissa (time).

mechanism so contraction occurs without change in length (isometrics) and when the muscles fiber contracts **isometrically, the tension developed is propotional to the number of cross linkages between** actin and myosin molecules. When muscle is stretched overlap between actin and myosin is reduced, conversely, when the muscles is shorter than resting length, distance the thin filaments can move is reduced.

(Pg. 71, 73)

5. Gap juctions:

A. Are absent in cardiac muscle

B. Are present but of little functional importance in cardiac muscle

C. Are present and provide the pathway for rapid spread of excitation from one cardiac muscle fiber to another

D. Are absent in smooth muscle

E. Connect the sarcotubular system to individual skeletal cells

Ans. (C)

Explanation:

Cell membranes are joined by many gap junctions through which ions, sugars, AA and other solutes with molecular weight up to about 1000 can pass. These junctions thus permit rapid propagation of electrical activity from cell to cell and use exchange of various chemical messengers,thus acting as low resistance bridges.They permit cardiac muscle to function as it if were a syncytium, even though no protoplasmic bridges are present between cells.The T system in cardiac muscle is located at the Z lines rather then at the A-I junction,where it is located in mammalian skeletal muscle.

(Guyton, 11th Ed.,Pg. 92, 93, 559, 771)

6. Duchenne's muscular dystrophy is caused by:

A. Reduced production of ATP
B. Mutation of the genes for Na+/Cl- channels
C. Absence of dystrophin
D. Alteration in the structure of dystrophin

Ans. (C)

Explanation:

Duchenne's muscular dystrophy is a serious from a dystrophy in which the dystrophin protein is absent from muscles. It is X-linked and usually fatal by the age of 30.

- Mutations in genes that code for enzymes involved in the metablism of carbohydrates, fats and proteins to CO_2 and H_2O in muscle and the production of ATP cause metabolic myopathies (**Mc Ardle's syndrome**).
- In **Myotonia**, muscle relaxation is prolonged after voluntary contraction. They are due to abnormal genes on chromosome 7, 17/19 which produce abnormalities of Na+/Ca^{+2} channels.

Beckers muscular dystropy: Dystrophin in present but altered or reduced in amount.

Limb-girdle muscular dystropy: Associated with mutation of the genes coding for the sarcoglycans or other components of the dystrophin-glycoprotein complex. *(Pg. 77)*

7. Amount of dystrophin at neuromuscular junction is:

A. Greater than utrophin at neuromuscular junction

B. Same as the amount of utrophin at neuromuscular junction

C. Less than the amount of utrophin at neuromuscular junction.

Ans. (C)

Explanation:

At neuromuscular junction (NMJ), dystrophin is replaced by utrophin, similar protein that is coded by a different gene.

8. Excitably of uterine smooth muslce after administration of progesterone is:

A. Greater than excitability of uterine smooth muscle after administration of estrogen

B. Same as excitability of uterine smooth muscle after administration of estrogen

C. Less than excitability of uterine smooth muscle after administration of estrogen

Ans. (C)

Explanation:

One of the factors responsible for onset of labor is increase in circulating estrogens. This makes the uterus more excitable while progesterone has a quieting effect on the uterus.

(Pg. 436)

Chapter 4 Synaptic and Junctional Transmission

1. **Which of the following is not found in appreciable quantities in postganglionic sympathetic neurons?**
   A. L-Dopa
   B. Dopamine
   C. Norepinephrine
   D. Histamine
   E. Acetylcholine

Ans. (D)

Explanation:

- Histaminergic neurons have their cell bodies in the tuberomamillary nucleus of posterior hypothalamus. Histamine is also found in cells of gastric mucosa and in heparin containing cells called mast cells that are plentiful in anterior and posterior lobes of pituitary glands.
- Acetylcholine (Ach) is released at anatomically sympa-thetic post-ganglionic neurons that innervate sweat glands, blood vessels in skeletal muscles and produce vasodilation when stimulated (**Sympathetic vasodilator nerves**). Nor-epinephrine, dopamine are catecholamines at post-ganglionic sympathetic neurons.

(Pg. 107, 224)

2. **Fast inhibitory postsynaptic potentials (IPSPs):**
   A. Are a consequence of decreased Cl^- conductance
   B. Occur in skeletal muscle
   C. Can be produced by an increase in Na^+ conductance
   D. Can be produced by an increase in Ca^{2+} conductance

E. Interact with other fast and slow potentials to move the membrane potential of the postsynaptic neuron toward or away from the firing level

Ans. (E)

Explanation:

The decreased excitability of nerve cell during IPSP is due to movement of membrane potential away from firing level.

- It can be produced by localized increase in Cl^- transport, it can also be produced by opening of K^+ channels, with movement of K^+ out of postsynaptic cell. In addition, they can be produced by closure of Na^+ or Ca^{+2} channels. *(Pg. 90)*

3. Initiation of an action potential in skeletal muscle by stimulating its motor nerve:

A. Requires spatial facilitation
B. Requires temporal facilitation
C. Is inhibited by a high concentration of Ca^{+2} at the neuromuscular junction
D. Requires the release of norepinephrine
E. Requires the release of acetylcholine

Ans. (E)

Explanation:

Transmission from nerve to muscle resembles chemical synaptic transmission from one neuron to another. The NMJ, the specialized area where a motor nerve terminates on a skeletal muscle fiber, is the site of a stereotyped transmission process, where Ach is released.

(Pg. 85)

4. Which of the following is a ligand-gated ion channel?

A. VIP receptor
B. Norepinephrine receptor

C. $GABA_A$ receptor
D. $GABA_B$ receptor
E. Metabotropic glutamine receptor

Ans. (C)

Explanation:

Three types of GABA receptors have been described. $GABA_A$, $GABA_B$ and $GABA_C$. The $GABA_A$ and $GABA_B$ receptors are widely distributed in CNS, while $GABA_C$ receptors are found exclusivey in retina. $GABA_A$ and $GABA_C$ receptors are ion channels (Cl^-) made up of 5 subunits surrounding a pore. The $GABA_B$ receptors are metabotropic and are coupled to heterotrimeric G proteins that increase conductance in:

- K^+ channels.
- Inhibits adenylyl cyclase.
- Inhibits Ca^{+2} influx.

5. Which of the following is most likely not to be involved in production of LTP?

A. NO
B. Ca^{2+}
C. NMDA receptors
D. Membrane hyperpolarization
E. Membrane depolarization

Ans. (D)

Explanation:

- NMDA receptors (N-methyl-D-asparatate) concentration is high in hippocampus. They are ionotropic receptors for **glutamate**. Blockade of these receptors prevent, LTP (long-term potentation), (a long-lasting facilitation of transmission in neural pathways following a brief period of high frequency stimulation. Thus these receptors may well be involved in memory and learning. NMDA receptor permits passage of relatively large amounts of Ca^{+2}.

- NO may be the signal by which post ganglionic neurons communicate with presynaptic endings in LTP and long-term depression.

6. Which of the following synaptic transmitters is not a peptide, polypeptide or protein?

A. Substance P
B. Met-enkephalin
C. β-Endorphin
D. Serotonin
E. Dynorphin

Ans. (D)

Explanation:

- Serotonin is formed in the body by hydroxylation and decarboxylation of the essential AA tryptophan.
- Enkephalins are pentapeptides (met-enkephalin, leuenkephalin, endorphin, dynorphin).

(Pg. 106)

7. Activation of which of the following receptors would be expected to decrease anxiety?

A. Nicotinic receptors
B. Glutamate receptors
C. $GABA_A$ receptors
D. Glucocorticoid receptors
E. α_1-Adrenergic receptors

Ans. (C)

Explanation:

Increase in Cl^- conductance produced by $GABA_A$ receptors (Q. 4) is potentiated by benzodiazepines, drugs that have marked anti-anxiety activity and are also effective muscle relaxants, anticonvulsants and sedatives.

8. Which of the following receptors is coupled to a heterotrimeric G protein?

A. Glycine receptor
B. $GABA_B$ receptor
C. Nicotinic acetylcholine receptor at myoneural junction
D. $5\text{-}HT_3$ receptor
E. ANP receptor

Ans. (B)

Explanation:

- **Glycine receptor** is a Cl^- channel. It is a pentamer made up of 2 subunits. *(Pg. 101)*
- **Nicotinic acetylcholine receptors** are members of a superfamily of ligand-gated ion channels that also includes the $\mathbf{GABA_A}$ and **glycine receptors** and **some of glutamate receptors.**
- **ANP receptor:** Both span cell membrane and have cytoplasmic domains that are guanylyl cyclases. *(Pg. 461)*

9. Which of the following would not be expected to enhance noradrenergic transmission?

A. A drug that increases the entry of arginine into neurons
B. A drug that increas tyrosine hydroxylase activity
C. A drug that enhances dopamine β-hydroxylase activity
D. A drug that inhibits monoamine oxidase
E. A drug that inhibits norepinephrine reuptake

Ans. (A)

Explanation:

- Norepinephrine (NE) secreting neurons are properly called **noradrenergic neurons** although the term **adrenergic neurons** is also applied. The principal **catecholamines** found in the body are **NE, E (epinephrine)**

and dopamine. They are formed by decarboxylation and hydroxylation of the amino acid **tyrosine.** Tyrosine is transported into catecholamine secreting neurons and adrenal medullary cells by a concentrating mechanism. It is converted to dopa and then to dopamine in the cytoplasm of the cells by **tyrosine hydroxylase** and **dopa decarboxylase respectively.**

(Pg. 101,102)

Phenylalanine
↓Phenylalanine hydroxylase
Tyrosine
↓Tyrosine hydroxylase
Dopa (dihydroxy phenylalanine)
↓aminoacid decarboxylase
Dopamine
↓dopamine-β-hydroxylase
Norepinephrine
↓phenylethanolamine-N-methyltransferase (PNMT)
Epinephrine

Both E and NE are metabolized to biologically inactive products by **oxidation** (by MAO monoamine oxidase) and **methylation** (COMT) (Catechol-O-methyl transferase).

(Pg. 103)

10. Number of times a β_2-adrenergic receptor spans the cell membrane is:

A. Greater than the number of times an M_1 muscarinic acetylcholine receptor spans the cell membrane

B. Same as the number of times an M_1 muscarinic acetylcholine receptor spans the cell membrane

C. Less than the number of times an M_1 muscarinic acetylcholine receptor spans the cell membrane

Ans. (B)

Explanation:

Same as number of times an M_1 muscarinic acetylcholine receptor spans the cell membrane.

Both α and β receptors are typical serpentine receptors linked to G proteins. They are closely related to the cloned receptors for dopamine, serotonin and to muscarinic acetylcholine receptors. *(Pg. 103)*

11. Amount of gephyrin in postsynaptic density is:

A. Greater than the amount of gephyrin in presynaptic active zone
B. Same as the amount of gephyrin in presynaptic active zones
C. Less than the amount of gephyrin in presynaptic active zones

Ans. (A)

Explanation:

$GABA_A$ receptors are associated with protein **gephyrin,** which also binds glycine receptors. In case of $GABA_A$ receptors, the binding protein **gephyrin** is located in clumps in the postsynaptic membrane. With activity, the free receptors move rapidly to the **gephyrin** and bind to it, creating membrane clusters. Gephyrin binding slows and restricts their further movement.

UNIT II. PHYSIOLOGY OF NERVE AND MUSCLE CELLS

Chapter 5 Initiation of Impulses in Sense Organs

1. **Pacinian corpuscles are:**
   A. A type of temperature receptor
   B. Usually innervated by Aδ nerve fibers
   C. Rapidly adapting touch receptors
   D. Slowly adapting touch receptors
   E. Pain receptors

Ans. (C)

Explanation:

Pacinian corpuscles are **touch** receptors. **Light touch** appears to have **rapidly adapting** receptors, while **spindle** and **nociceptor** input is **slowly adapting.** *(Pg. 123-124)*
Meissner's and Pacinian corpuscles are rapidly adapting touch receptors.

2. **Adaptation to a sensory stimulus produces:**
   A. A diminished sensation when other types of sensory stimuli are withdrawn
   B. A more intense sensation when a given stimulus is applied repeatedly
   C. A sensation localized to the hand when the nerves of the brachial plexus are stimulated
   D. A diminished sensation when a given stimulus is applied repeatedly over time
   E. A decreased firing rate in the sensory nerve from the receptor when one's attention is directed to another matter

Ans. (D)

Explanation:

When a maintained stimulus of constant strength is applied to a receptor, the frequency of AP (action potential) in its sensory nerve declines over time. This phenomenon is known as **adaptation or desensitization.**

(Pg. 124)

3. **Which of the following sensations is not generated by impulses initiated in naked nerve endings?**
   - A. Touch
   - B. Pain
   - C. Cold
   - D. Tickle
   - E. Proprioception

Ans. (E)

Explanation:

Proprioception ("body image") is actually synthesized from information coming not only from the receptors in and around joints but also from cutaneous touch and pressure receptors.

(Pg. 122)

4. **In which of the following is the frequency of stimulation not linearly related to the strength of the sensation felt?**
   - A. Sensory area of the cerebral cortex
   - B. Specific projection nuclei of the thalamus
   - C. Lateral spirithalamic tract
   - D. Dorsal horn
   - E. Cutaneous receptors

Ans. (E)

Explanation:

- It was earlier believed that **magnitude of sensation felt α log of intensity of stimulus.**
  (Weber-Fechnar Law)
- But now there are many constants between them e.g.:
  $R = K S^A$

where

R=Sensation felt

S= Intensity of stimulus

K and A are constants. That is relation between direct stimulation of a sensory nerve and sensation felt is linear, however the frequency of AP generation in a sensory nerve fiber is also related to intensity of initiating stimulus by power function, consequently it appears that for any given sensory modality, the relation between sensation and stimulus intensity is determined primarily by the properties of the peripheral receptors themselves. *(Pg. 126)*

5. Which of the following receptors and sense organs are incorrectly paired?

A. Rods and cones: eye
B. Receptors sensitive to sodium: taste buds
C. Hair cells: olfactory mucous membranes
D. Receptors sensitive to stretch: carotid sinus
E. Glomus cells: carotid body

Ans. (C)

Explanation:

Hair cells are receptors for **Ear**.

while for OMM (**Olfactory mucous membrane**), receptors are **olfactory neurons**.

(Pg. 122)

6. Which of the following sensations is most subject to facilitation and inhibition in the central nervous system?

A. Touch
B. Warmth
C. Pain
D. Hearing
E. Taste

Ans. (C)

Explanation:

Central inhibition plays important role in perception of pain sensation.

7. **Which of the following does not contain cation channels that are activated by mechanical distortion, producing depolarization?**

A. Olfactory neurons
B. Pacinian corpuscles
C. Hair cells in cochlea
D. Hair cells in semicircular canals
E. Hair cells in utricle

Ans. (A)

Explanation:

Each olfactory receptor is a neuron, OMM (Olfactory mucus membrane) might contain one or more odorent binding proteins (OBP) that concentrate the odorants and transfer them to the receptors.

(Pg. 187)

8. **Amptitude of generator potential with weak stimulus is:**

A. Greater than amplitude of generator potential with strong stimulus
B. Same as amplitude of generator potential with strong stimulus
C. Less than amplitude of generator potential with strong stimulus

Ans. (C)

Explanation:

As the pressure is increased, magnitude of receptor potential increases. As pressure is further increased generator potential becomes even larger and sensory nerve fires repetitively (studied using pacinian corpuscles)

(Pg. 123)

9. Amplitude of action potentials in sensory nerve with weak stimulus:

A. Greater than the amplitude of action potentials in sensory nerve with strong stimulus

B. Same as the amplitude of action potentials in sensory nerve with strong stimulus

C. Less than the amplitude of action potentials in sensory nerve with strong stimulus

Ans. (B)

Explanation:

Action potential (AP) occurs with a constant amplitude and form regardless of the strength of stimulus if the stimulus is at or above threshold intensity. *(Pg. 54-55)*

UNIT III. NERVOUS SYSTEM

Chapter 6 Reflexes

1. The inverse stretch reflex:

A. Has a lower threshold than the stretch reflex

B. Is a monosynaptic reflex

C. Is a disynaptic reflex with a single interneuron inserted between the afferent and efferent limbs

D. Is a polysynaptic reflex with many interneurons inserted between the afferent and efferent limbs

E. Requires the discharge of central neurons that release acetylcholine

Ans. (C)

Explanation:

Inverse stretch reflex is a disynaptic reflex with a single interneuron inserted between the afferent and efferent limbs. Upto a point, the harder a muscle is stretcted, the stronger is the reflex contraction. However,when the tension becomes great enough, contraction suddenly ceases and muscle relaxes. This relaxation in response to strong stretch is called inverse stretch reflex/ autogenic inhibition.

- **Receptor** for **inverse stretch reflex** is **Golgi tendon organ**.

(Pg. 133)

See Flow Chart on the next page

Pathway for stretch reflex and inverse stretch reflex

Stretch	**Stretch**
↓	↓
Stimulation of muscle spindle	Stimulation of Golgi tendon organ
↓	↓
Impulses pass up the Ia fiber	Impulses pass up the Ib fibers
↓	↓
Excitation of motor neuron	Activation of interneuron
↓	↓
Contraction of muscle	Release of inhibitory mediator **glycine**
	↓
	Hyperpolarization
	↓
	Relaxation of muscle

2. **When γ motor neuron discharge increases at the same time as α motor neuron discharge to muscle:**
   - **A.** Prompt inhibition of discharge in spindle Ia afferents takes place
   - **B.** The contraction of the muscle is prolonged
   - **C.** The muscle will not contract
   - **D.** The number of impulses in spindle Ia afferents is smaller than when α discharge alone is increased
   - **E.** The number of impulses in spindle Ia afferents is greater than when α discharge alone is increased

Ans. (E)

Explanation:

There is considerable evidence of increased γ

efferent discharge along with the increased discharge of the α motor neurons that initiates muscle movements. Because of this α-γ linkage, the spindle shortens with the muscle and spindle discharge may continue throughout the contraction. In this way, the spindle remains capable of responding to stretch and reflexly adjusting motor neuron discharge throughout the contraction. *(Pg. 132)*

3. Which of the following is not characteristic of a reflex action?

A. Modification by impulses from various parts of the central nervous system
B. May involve simultaneous contraction of some muscles and relaxation of others
C. May involve either somatic or visceral responses but never both simultaneously
D. Always involves transmission across at least one synapse
E. Frequency occurs without conscious perception

Ans. (C)

Explanation:

Reflex can be monosynaptic (stretch reflex e.g. knee jerk) or polysynaptic (Withdrawal reflex). In both types, but specially in polysynaptic reflex arcs, activity is modified by spatial and temporal facilitation, occlusion, subliminal fringe effects and other effects. Muscle spindles and Golgi tendon organs also apprise the higher motor control centers of instantaneous changes taking place in the muscles e.g. Dorsal spinocerebellar tracts carry instantaneous information from both muscles spindles and Golgi tendon organs directly to cerebrum, additional pathway transmit similar information into reticular areas of brainstem and cerebral cortex.

(Guyton, 11th Ed., Pg. 680)

When central excitatory state is marked, excitatory impulses irradiate not only to many somatic areas of spinal cord but also to autonomic areas (**Mass reflex).** *(Pg. 137)*

4. **Withdrawal reflexes are *not*:**

A. Initiated by nociceptive stimuli
B. Prepotent
C. Prolonged if the stimulus is strong
D. Affected by transection of the spinal cord
E. Dependent on local sign for their exact pattern

Ans. (D)

Explanation:

- Withdrawal reflexes are polysynaptic reflexes that occur in response to a noxious and painful stimulation of skin/subcutaneous tissues and muscles. They are **prepotent** i.e. they preempt the spinal pathways from any other reflex activity taking place at the moment.
- Due to **after discharge** i.e. prolonged response due to prolonged, repeated firing of motor neurons is due to continued bombardment of motor neurons by impulses arriving by complicated and circuitious polysynaptic pathways.
- The exact response depends on the location of stimulus (**local sign**).
- Once the spinal reflexes begin to reappear after spinal shock, their threshold steadily drops. In chronically quadriplegic humans, the threshold of the withdrawal reflex is especially low. *(Pg. 209)*

Chapter 7 Cutaneous, Deep and Visceral Sensation

1. **The distance by which two touch stimuli must be separated to be perceived as two separate stimuli is greatest on:**
   A. The lips
   B. The palm of the hand
   C. The back of the scapula
   D. The dorsum of the hand
   E. The tips of the fingers

Ans. (C)

Explanation:

Touch receptors are **most numerous** in the skin of the **fingers** and **lips** and relatively scare in the skin of the trunk. The minimal distance by which two touch stimuli must be separated to be perceived as separate is called two-point threshold. Points on the back must be separated by 65 mm or more before they can be distinguished as separate, whereas in the fingers two stimuli can be resolved if they are separated by as little as 3 mm. *(Pg. 141-147)*

2. **A 49-year-old blond woman has diffuse, severe loss of vibration sensitivity. Which of the following tests would give you the most information about the cause of her loss?**
   A. X-rays of her spine
   B. Determination of her reflex reaction time
   C. Measurement of the protein content of her cerebrospinal fluid
   D. A biopsy of her gastric mucosa
   E. A complete urinalysis

Ans. (D)

Explanation:

Receptors involved for vibration sense are touch, especially **pacinian corpuscles.** The impulses responsible for the **vibrating sensation** are carried in **dorsal columns**. Degeneration of this part of the spinal cord occurs in poorly controlled **diabetes, pernicious anemia and some vitamin deficiencies.** Elevation of the threshold for vibratory stimuli is an early symptom of this degeneration. *(Pg. 147)*

3. **Stimulation of which of the following might be expected to produce itching?**

A. Dorsal root C fibers
B. B fibers in peripheral nerves
C. Dorsal columns of the spinal cord
D. Touch receptors
E. Motor fibers in the ventral roots of the spinal nerves

Ans. (A)

Explanation:

Itching is due to dorsal root C fibers stimulation. *(Pg. 147)*

4. **Visceral pain:**

A. Shows relatively rapid adaptation
B. Is mediated by B fibers in the dorsal roots of the spinal nerves
C. Can sometimes be relieved by applying an irritant to the skin
D. Most closely resembles "fast pain" produced by noxious stimulation of the skin
E. Can be produced by marked and prolonged stimulation of touch receptors

Ans. (C)

Explanation:

Afferent fibers from visceral structures reach CNS via sympathetic and parasympathetic pathways. Their cell bodies are located in the dorsal roots and the homologous cranial nerve ganglia. Specifically, there are visceral afferents in the **VII, IX, X nerves** in the **thoracic** and **upper lumbar dorsal roots and in sacral roots.** Use of counter irritants helps to relieve pain due to primarily inhibition of pain pathways in the dorsal horn gate by stimulation of large diameter **touch-pressure afferents.** *(Pg. 145)*

5. **An anterolateral cordotomy is performed that produces relief of pain in the right leg. It is effective because it interrupts the:**

A. Left dorsal column
B. Left ventral spinothalamic tract
C. Right lateral spinothalamic tract
D. Left lateral spinothalamic tract
E. Right corticospinal tract

Ans. (D)

Explanation:

Spinothalamic tract (Ventral and lateral) cross midline where they carry **touch, pain** and **temperature** sensations to opposite side of body.

6. **Which of the following does not exert an analgesic effect?**

A. Morphine
B. Cholinergic antagonists
C. Adrenergic antagonists
D. Substance P antagonists
E. Anandamide

Ans. (B)

Explanation:

Cholinergic agoinst (e.g. epibatidine) are found to be a potent nonopoid analgesic agents and their effects are blocked by cholinergic blocking drugs.

- Cannabinoids **(anandamide)** are produced endogenously and have definite analgesic effects.

- There are anandamide-containing neurons in periaqueductal grey and other areas concerned with pain.
- **Substance 'P'** is said to be released during muscle contraction which causes pain when its local concentration is high. *(Pg. 143)*

7. A man loses his right hand in a farm accident. Four years later, he has episodes of severe pain in the missing hand (phantom limb pain). A detailed PET scan study of his cerebral cortex might be expected to show:

A. Expansion of the right hand area in his right somatic sensory area I (SI)
B. Expansion of the right hand area in his left SI
C. A metabolically inactive spot where his hand area in his left SI would normally be
D. Projection of fibers from neighboring sensory areas into the right hand area of his right SI
E. Projection of fibers from neighboring sensory areas into the right hand area of his left SI

Ans. (E)

Explanation:

Due to cortical representation of neighboring areas into the cortical area that was formerly occupied by the representation of the amputated hand. Conversely, if the cortical area representing a body part is removed, the somatosensory map of that part of body moves to the surrounding cortex. The explanation of these shifts appears to be that cortical connections of sensory units to the cortex have extensive convergence and divergence with connections that can become weak with disuse and strong with use. This is called **cortical plasticity** which occurs not only with input from cutaneous receptors but also with input in other sensory systems e.g. vision and hearing. *(Pg. 141)*

8. **Causalgia is:**

   A. Associated with loss of hair in the affected area
   B. Abolished by sectioning the sensory nerves in the affected area
   C. Relieved by drugs that block glycine receptors
   D. Relieved by drugs that block α_1 adrenergic receptors
   E. Relieved by drugs that block muscarinic cholinergic receptors

Ans. (D)

Explanation:

In **causalgia (nerve injury)**, there is spontaneous, burning pain which occurs long after seemingly trivial injuries. The pain is often accompanied by **hyperalgesia** and **allodynia. Reflex sympathetic dystrophy** is often present as well. In this condition the skin in the affected area is thin and shiny and there is increased hair growth. Research shows nerve injury leads to sprouting and eventual overgrowth of noradrenergic sympathetic nerve fibers into the dorsal root ganglia of sensory nerves from the injured area. So α-adrenergic blockage produces relief.

9. **Rate of conduction in afferent neurons from cold receptors is:**

   A. Greater than rate of conduction in afferent neurons from pressure receptors
   B. Same as rate of conduction in afferent neurons from pressure receptors
   C. Less than rate of conduction in afferent neurons from pressure receptors

Ans. (C)

Explanation:

Aβ fibers (large myelinated fibers) carry **pressure** sensation at 30-70 m/s while **cold** sensation is carried primarily by small unmyelinated **C** fibers at 0.5-2 m/s.

10. Effects of parietal lobe lesions on stereognosis are:

A. Greater than effect of frontal lobe lesions on stereognosis

B. Same as effect of frontal lobe lesions on stereognosis

C. Less than effect of frontal lobe lesions on stereognosis

Ans. (A)

Explanation:

Impaired **stereognosis** is there when there is lesion in the parietal lobe posterior to the postcentral gyrus.

Chapter 8 Vision

1. **If the principal focal distance of a lens is 0.75 m, its refractive power is:**
   A. 0.25 diopter
   B. 0.75 diopter
   C. 1.0 diopter
   D. 1.33 diopters
   E. 10.3 diopters

Ans. (D)

Explanation:

R.P. = 1/focal length (m)
Therefore
R.P. = 1/0.75 m = 1.33D

2. **Visual accommodation involves:**
   A. Increased tension on the lens ligaments
   B. A decrease in the curvature of the lens
   C. Relaxation of the sphincter muscle of the iris
   D. Contraction of the ciliary muscle
   E. Increased intraocular pressure

Ans. (D)

Explanation:

When ciliary muscle is relaxed, parallel light rays striking the optically normal (emmetropic) eye are brought to a focus on the retina. When gaze is directed at a near object, ciliary muscle contracts, leading to increase in curvature of lens called as **Accommodation**.

(Pg. 153)

3. **The fovea of the eye:**
   A. Has the lowest light threshold
   B. Is the region of highest visual acuity

C. Contains only red and green cones
D. Contains only rods
E. Is situated over the head of the optic nerve

Ans. (B)

Explanation:

The fovea of the eye is a thinned out, rod-free portion of the retina that is present in humans and other primates. In it, the cones are densely packed and each synapses to a single bipolar cell, which in turn synapses on a single ganglion cell, providing a direct pathway to the brain. There are few overlying cells and no blood vessels. Consequently, the fovea is the point where visual acuity is greatest.

(Pg. 149)

4. Which of the following parts of the eye has the greatest concentration of rods?

A. Ciliary body
B. Iris
C. Optic disk
D. Fovea
E. Parafoveal region

Ans. (E)

Explanation:

In extra foveal portions of the retina, rods predominate and there is good deal of convergence. *(Pg. 150)*

5. The following events that occur in rods in response to light are listed in random sequence:

1. Activation of transduction
2. Decreased release of synaptic transmitter
3. Structural changes in rhodopsin
4. Closure of Na^+ channels
5. Decrease in intracellular cGMP

What is the sequence in which they normally occur?

A. 2, 1, 3, 5, 4
B. 1, 2, 3, 5, 4
C. 5, 3, 1, 4, 2
D. 3, 1, 5, 4, 2
E. 3, 1, 4, 5, 2

Ans. **(D)**

Explanation:

Phototransduction (i.e. conversion of one form of energy to another) in rods and cones is as below:

(Pg. 159)

Incident light
↓
Structural change in retinene$_1$ of photopigment
↓
Conformational change of photopigment
↓
Activation of transducin
↓
Activation of phosphodiesterase
↓
Decreased intracellular cGMP
↓
Closure of Na^+ channels
↓
Hyperpolarization
↓
Decreased release of synaptic transmitter
↓
Response in bipolar cells and other neural elements

6. Vitamin A is a precursor for the synthesis of:

A. Somatostatin
B. Retinene$_1$
C. The pigment of the iris
D. Scotopsin
E. Aqueous humor

Ans. **(B)**

Explanation:

Photosensitive compounds in the rods and cones of the eyes of humans and most other mammals are made up of a protein called an opsin and retinene$_1$ (the aldehyde of vitamin A_1). **(Retinene$_2$ is found in the eyes of some animal species).**

7. **Abnormal color vision is 20 times more common in men than women because most cases are caused by an abnormal:**
   A. Dominant gene on the Y chromosome
   B. Recessive gene on the Y chromosome
   C. Dominant gene on the X chromosome
   D. Recessive gene on the X chromosome
   E. Recessive gene on chromosome 22

Ans. (D)

Explanation:

Color blindness/abnormal color vision is inherited as recessive and X-linked disorders, i.e., they are due to an abnormal gene on the X-chromosome.

8. **Which of the following is not involved in color vision?**
   A. Activation of a pathway that signals differences between S cone responses and the sum of L and M cone responses
   B. Geniculate layers 3-6
   C. P pathway
   D. Area V3A of visual cortex
   E. Area V8 of visual cortex

Ans. (D)

Explanation:

Primary visual cortex (V1) projects to many parts of the occipital lobes and other parts of the brain. These are often identified by numbers (V2, V3) or by letters (LO, MT, etc). Area V8 appears to be uniquely **concerned with color vision in humans.** *(Pg. 161)*

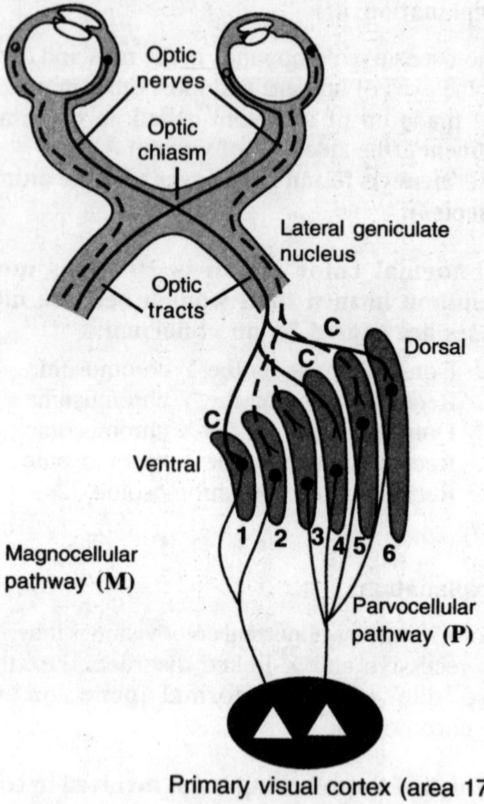

Primary visual cortex (area 17)

Color is mediated by ganglion cells that subtract or add input from one type of cone to input from another type.

Ganglion cells

↓

LGN (lateral geniculate nucleus)

↓ 3 Neural pathway

Red-green pathway (L and M cones) | Blue-yellow pathway (L and M cones) | Luminance pathway (L and M cones)

↓

Blobs and deep portion of layer 4C of V1

↓

V8 Converts color input into sensation of color.

Based on wavelength of light, cones are maximum sensitive, they are divided into short wave (S), middle wave (M) and long wave (L) cones.

(Pg. 165)

9. Number of action potentials (AP) in right visual cortex after stimulation of medial half of right retina is:

A. Greater than number of AP in left visual cortex after stimulation of medial half of right retina

B. Same as number of AP in left visual cortex after stimulation of medial half of right retina

C. Less than number of AP in left visual cortex after stimulation of medial half of right retina

Ans. (C)

Explanation:

Half of the fibers in each optic tract after passing the optic chiasma are derived from one eye and half from the other eye, representing corresponding points on the two retinas. However, the signals from the two eyes are kept apart in the **dorsal lateral geniculate nucleus (LGN).** This nucleus is composed of six nuclear layers. **LGN II, III and V layers**→receive signals from lateral (1/2) half of the **ipsilateral** retina, while **LGN I, IV, VI**→receive signals from the medial half of the retina of the **opposite** side.

(Guyton, 11th Ed., Pg. 640)

The respective retinal areas of the 2 eyes connect with neurons that are superimposed over one another in the paired layers and similar parallel transmission is preserved all the way to the visual cortex.

LGN (Visual Cortex)

Layer II, III, V	Layer I, IV, VI
↓	↓
Lateral ½ of ipsilateral retina	Medial ½ of opposite retina

Chapter 9 Hearing and Equilibrium

1. Sound intensity is measured in:

A. Diopters
B. Daltons
C. Torrs
D. Decibels
E. Pounds

Ans. (D)

Explanation:

Sound **intensity** is measured in decibels.

Number of dB $= 10 \log \frac{\textbf{intensity of sound}}{\text{intensity of standard sound}}$

Sound **intensity** is proportionate to the square of sound pressure

Number of dB $= 20 \log \frac{\textbf{pressure of sound}}{\text{pressure of standard sound}}$

0-140 dB range is from threshold pressure to a pressure that is potentially damaging to the organ of corti actually represents a 10 million fold variation in sound pressure. *(Pg. 177)*

2. In humans, the primary auditory cortex is located in the:

A. Limbic system
B. Posterior part of the occipital lobe
C. Posterior part of the parietal lobe
D. Postcentral gyrus
E. Superior part of the temporal lobe

Ans. (E)

Explanation:

Primary **auditory cortex (area 41) is located in superior part of the temporal lobe.**

3. Post rotatory nystagmus is caused by continued movement of:

A. Aqueous humor over the ciliary body in the eye
B. Cerebrospinal fluid over the parts of the brain-stem that contain the vestibular nuclei
C. Endolymph in the semicircular canals, with consequent bending of the cupula and stimulation of hair cells
D. Endolymph toward the helicotrema
E. Perilymph over hair cells that have their processes embedded in the tectorial membrane

Ans. (C)

Explanation:

Semicircular canals are concerned with equilibrium. Receptors in semicircular canals (hair cells), detect **rotational acceleration**. Post rotatory nystagmus is due to continued movement of endolymph in the canals with consequent bending of cupula and stimulation of hair cells. *(Pg. 174, 184)*

4. The basilar membrane of the cochlea:

A. Is unaffected by movement fluid in the scala vestibuli
B. Covers the oval window and the round window
C. Vibrates in a pattern determined by the form of the travelling wave in the fluids in the cochlea
D. Is under tension
E. Vibrates when the body is subjected to linear acceleration

Ans. (C)

Explanation:

The movements of the footplate of the stapes set up a series of travelling waves in the perilymph of the scala vestibuli. The bony walls of the scala vestibuli are rigid, but Reissner's membrane is flexible. The basilar membrane is not under tension and it also is readily depressed into the scala tympani by the peaks of waves into the scala vestibuli. Therefore, sound produces distortion of the basilar membrane and the site at which this distortion is maximal is determined by the frequency of sound wave.

(Pg. 179)

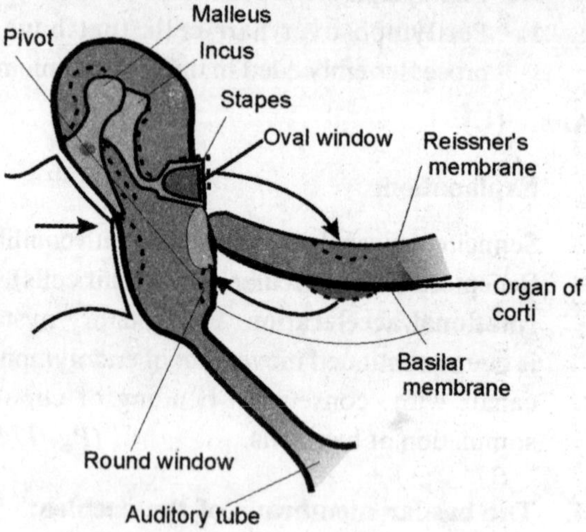

Representation of auditory ossicles and the way their movement translates movements of the tympanic membrane into a wave in the fluid of the inner ear. The wave is dissipated at the round window. Movement of ossicles, membranous labyrinth and round window are indicated by dashed lines.

5. **Some diseases damage the hair cells in the ear. When the damage to the outer hair cells is greater than the damage to the inner hair cells:**
   A. The perception of vertical acceleration is disrupted
   B. The K^+ concentration in endolymph is decreased

C. The K^+ concentration in perilymph is decreased
D. There is severe hearing loss
E. The affected hair cells fail to shorten when exposed to sound

Ans. (E)

Explanation:

Outer hairs cells respond to sound, like the inner hair cells, but depolarization makes them shorten and hyperpolarization makes them lengthen. This action somehow increases the amplitude and clarity of sounds.

(Pg. 180)

6. Which of the following are *incorrectly* paired?

A. Tympanic membrane: manubrium of malleus
B. Helicotrema: apex of cochlea
C. Foot plate of stapes: oval window
D. Otoliths: semicircular canals
E. Basement membrane: cochlea

Ans. (D)

Explanation:

Otoliths are present in utricle and saccule. They are crystals of calcium carbonate, they are also called otoconia/eardust, range from 3-19 μm in length in humans and are more dense than the endolymph. *(Pg. 173)*

7. The direction of nystagmus is vertical when a subject is rotated:

A. After warm water is put in one ear
B. With the head tipped backward
C. After cold water is put in both ears
D. With the head tipped sideways
E. After section of one vestibular nerve

Ans. (D)

Explanation:

The characteristic jerky movement of the eye observed at the start and end of a period of rotation is called nystagmus. Nystagmus is frequently horizontal (i.e. eyes move in a horizontal plane), but it can also be vertical, when the head is tipped sidewise during rotation, or rotatory when the head is tipped forward. *(Pg. 184)*

8. The human planum temporale is:

A. Concerned with auditory-visual coordination
B. Concerned with detection of liner acceleration
C. Concerned with localization of sound
D. Larger in the cerebral hemisphere than in the left
E. Generally larger in musicians with perfect pitch than in musicians without perfect pitch

Ans. (E)

Explanation:

A portion of the **posterior superior temporal gyrus known as planum temporale** is larger in left than in right cerebral hemisphere, particularly in right handed individuals. This area appears to be involved in language related auditory processing. It is even more larger than normal on the left side i.e. asymmetry is greater in musicians and others who have perfect pitch.

(Pg.181-182)

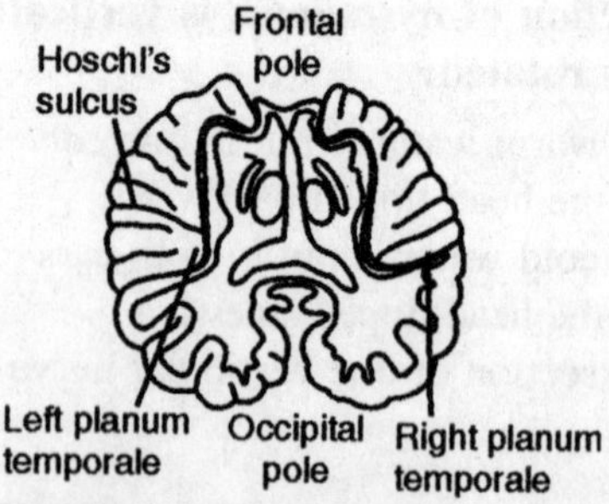

Left and right planum temporale in a brain sectioned horizontally along the plane of the sylvian fissure

9. **In the utricle, tip links in hair cells are involved in:**
   A. Formation of perilymph
   B. Depolarization of the stria vascularis
   C. Movements of the basement membrane
   D. Perception of sound
   E. Regulation of distortion-activated ion channels

Ans. (E)

Explanation:

Very fine process called tip links, tie the tip of each stereocilium to the side of its higher neighbour and at the junction are cation ion channels in the higher process that appear to be mechanically sensitive. When the shorter stereocilia are pushed toward the higher, the open time of these channels increases. K^+ and Ca^{+2} enter via channel, producing depolarization. *(Pg. 176)*

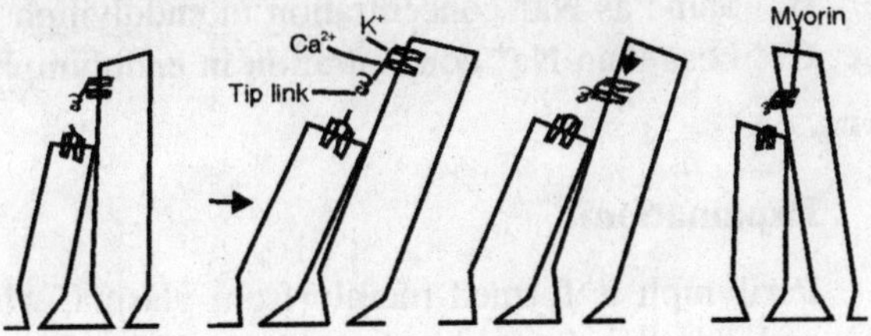

Role of tip links in the responses of hair cells

10. **A patient enters the hospital for evaluation of deafness. He is found to also have an elevated plasma renin, although his blood pressure is 118/75 mm Hg. Mutation of what single gene would be likely to explain these findings?**
    A. The gene for barttin
    B. The gene for Na^+ channel
    C. The gene for renin
    D. The gene for cystic fibrosis transmembrane conductance regulator
    E. The gene for tyrosine hydroxylase

Ans. (A)

Explanation:

Bartter's syndrome is due to defective transport in thick ascending limb, due to chronic Na^+ loss in the urine. The condition can be caused by loss of function mutation in the gene for **ClC-KbCl$^-$** channel or **barttin** that is necessary for normal function of ClC-KbCl$^-$ channels.

The stria vascularis in the inner ear is responsible for maintaining high K^+ concentration in scala media that is essential for normal hearing. It contains both ClC-Kb and ClC-KaCl$^-$ channels. So patients with Bartter's syndrome due to mutated barttin are deaf because both types of Cl$^-$l channels are barttin-dependent. *(Pg. 715)*

11. Na^+ concentration in perilymph is:

A. Greater than Na^+ concentration in endolymph
B. Same as Na^+ concentration in endolymph
C. Less than Na^+ concentration in endolymph

Ans. (A)

Explanation:

Perilymph is formed mainly from plasma, while endolymph is formed in the scala media by the stria vascularis and has a high concentration of K^+ and a low concentration of Na^+. This difference is due to:

1. Presence in the stria vascularis, a high concentration of Na^+-K^+ ATPase.
2. In addition, it appears that a unique electrogenic K^+ pump in scala media accounts for scala media +85mV (electrically positive) relative to scala vestibuli and scala media.

12. Maximum sound frequency audible to humans is:

A. Greater than maximum sound frequency **audible** to dogs

B. Same as maximum sound frequency **audible** to dogs
C. Less than maximum sound frequency **audible** to dogs

Ans. (C)

Explanation:

The sound frequencies audible to humans range from 20-20,000 cycles/sec. In other animals, e.g. bats and dogs much higher frequencies are audible. *(Pg. 178)*

13. Change in membrane potential when stereocilia of a saccular hair cell are pushed toward the kinocilium:

A. Greater than change in membrane potential when stereocilia of a saccular hair cell are pushed at a right angle to the kinocilium
B. Same as change in membrane potential when stereocilia of a saccular hair cell are pushed at a right angle to the kinocilium
C. Less than change in membrane potential when stereocilia of a saccular hair cell are pushed at a right angle to the kinocilium

Ans. (A)

Explanation:

The membrane potential of the hair cells is about ¯60 mV. When the stereocilia are pushed toward kinocilium, the membrane potential is decreased to about -50mV. When the bundle of the process is pushed in opposite direction the cell is hyperpolarized. Displacement in a direction perpendicular to this axis provides no change in membrane potential and displacing the process in directions that are intermediate between these two directions produces depolarization or hyperpolarization proportionate to the degree to which the direction is towards or away from the kinocilium. *(Pg. 176)*

Chapter 10 Smell and Taste

1. Impulses generated by olfactory receptors in the nasal mucous membrane:

A. Pass through the substantia nigra
B. Pass through the internal capsule
C. Are relayed to the olfactory cortex via the hypothalamus
D. Pass to the mitral cells and from there directly to the olfactory cortex
E. Pass to the mitral cells and from there to the olfactory cortex via the taste area

Ans. (D)

Explanation:

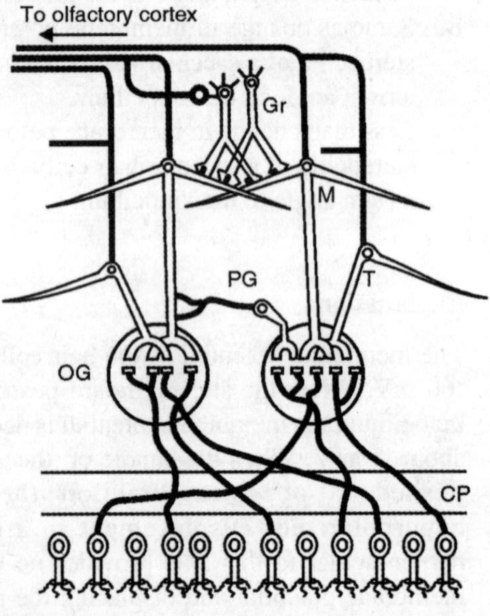

CP, cribriform plate
PG, perglomerular cell
M, mitral cell
T, tufted cell
Gr, granule cell

Basic neuronal circuits in olfactory bulb

Olfactory receptor cells with one type of odorant receptor project to one olfactory glomerulus (OG) and olfactory receptor cells with other type of odorant receptor project to a different olfactory glomerulus (OG). *(Pg. 186)*

2. Impulses generated in the taste buds of the tongue reach the cerebral cortex via the:

A. Thalamus
B. Internal capsule
C. Dorsal roots of the first cervical spinal nerves
D. Trochlear nerve
E. Hypoglossal nerve

Ans. (A)

Explanation:

(Pg.189)

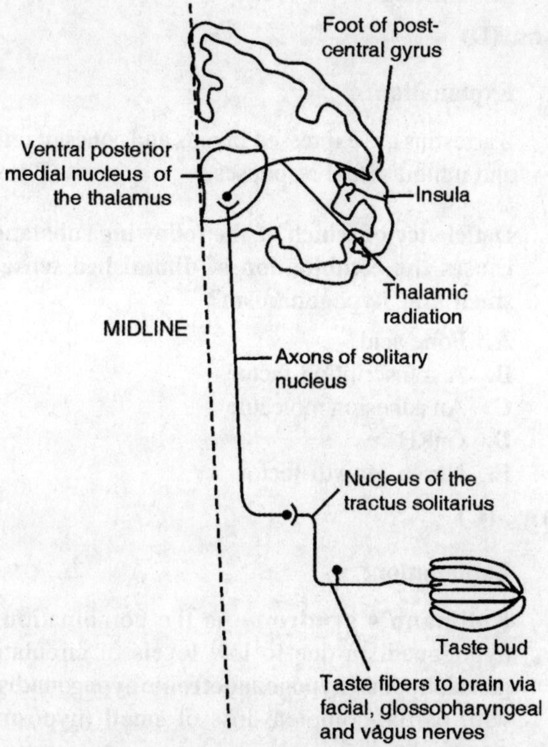

Diagram showing taste pathways

3. Which of the following senses is most strongly associated with aversive conditioning?

A. Pressure
B. Vision
C. Linear acceleration
D. Olfaction
E. Taste

Ans. (E)

4. Which of the following does not increase the ability to discriminate many different odors?

A. Many different receptors
B. Pattern of olfactory receptors activated by a given odorant
C. Projection of different mitral cell axons to different parts of the brain
D. High β-arrestin content in olfactory neurons
E. Sniffing

Ans. (D)

Explanation:

β arrestins are expressed in rods and cones of retina and inhibit visual responses. *(Pg. 97)*

5. Deficiency of which of the following substances causes the combination of diminished sense of smell and hypogonadism?

A. Folic acid
B. A transcription factor
C. An adhesion molecule
D. GnRH
E. Nerve growth factor

Ans. (C)

Explanation:

Kallmann's syndrome is the combination of hypogonadism due to low levels of circulating gonadotropins (**hypogonadotropic hypogonadism**) with partial/complete loss of smell (hyposmia/ anosmia).

Embryologically, GnRH neurons develop in the nose and migrate up the olfactory nerves and then through the brain to hypothalamus. If this migration is prevented by congenital abnormalities in the olfactory pathway, the GnRH neurons do not reach the hypothalamus and pubertal maturation of the gonads fails to occur. This syndrome is most common in men and cause in many cases is mutation of the KALIG 1 gene, a gene on the X chromosome that codes for what is apparently an adhesion molecule necessary for normal development of olfactory nerve on which the GnRH neurons migrate into the brain. *(Pg. 250)*

6. Which of the following are *incorrectly* paired?

A. α-Gusducin: sweet taste
B. α-Gusducin: bitter taste
C. Nucleus tractus solitarius: blood pressure
D. Insular cortex: smell
E. Ebner's glands: taste acuity

Ans. (D)

Explanation:

The insula is known to be activated by unpleasant tastes and this response evolved into activation of the area by faces showing disgust, so people who have selective lesions of left insula and putamen experienced difficulty recognizing disgust on the faces or in the voices of people the patient met. *(Pg. 260)*

7. Olfactory sensitivity in a 20-year-old woman is:

A. Greater than olfactory sensitivity in a 70-year-old woman
B. Same as olfactory sensitivity in a 70-year-old woman
C. Less than olfactory sensitivity in a 70-year-old woman

Ans. (A)

Explanation:

Olfactory thresholds increase with advancing age and > 75% of humans over age of 80 have an impaired ability to identify smells.

8. **Number of different G proteins involved in transduction of taste stimuli is:**
   - **A.** Greater than number of different G proteins involved in transduction of olfactory stimuli
   - **B.** Same as number of different G proteins involved in transduction of olfactory stimuli
   - **C.** Less than number of different G proteins involved in transduction of olfactory stimuli

Ans. (C)

Explanation:

More than 1% of genome is denoted to making odorant receptors. The genes for the receptor make up the largest gene family so far described in mammals. All the odorant receptors are coupled to heterotumeric G proteins.

(Pg. 187)

Chapter 11 Alert Behavior, Sleep and the Electrical Activity of the Brain

1. **In a healthy, alert adult sitting with the eyes closed, the dominant EEG rhythm observed with electrodes over the occipital lobes is:**
   - **A.** Delta (0.5-4 Hz)
   - **B.** Theta (4-7 Hz)
   - **C.** Alpha (8-13 Hz)
   - **D.** Beta (18-30 Hz)
   - **E.** Fast, irregular low-voltage activity

Ans. (C)

Explanation:

α-waves. In adult humans who are awake but at rest with the mind wandering and the eyes closed, the most prominent component of the EEG is fairly regular pattern of α-waves at:

- 8-12 Hz = Frequency.
- 50-100 μV = Amplitude.
- Most prominent over **parieto-occipital** area.

2. **The EEG record in figure below is characteristic of:**
   - **A.** Deep sleep
   - **B.** A learning response produced by a painful stimulus
   - **C.** REM sleep
   - **D.** A phychomotor seizure
   - **E.** An absence seizure

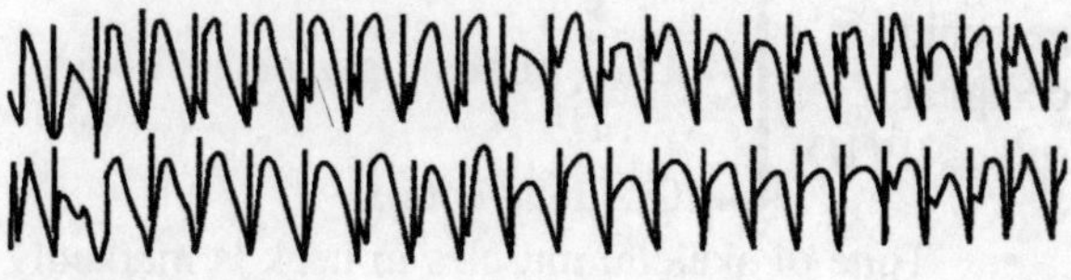

Ans. (E)

Explanation:

Absence (Petit Mal) seizures are one of the forms of generalized seizures characterized by a momentary loss of responsiveness. They are associated with 3/s doublets, each consisting of a typical spike and rounded wave.

3. **The electrical records in figure below are characteristic of:**

   A. Deep sleep
   B. General-onset seizures
   C. REM sleep
   D. Psychomotor seizures
   E. An absence seizure

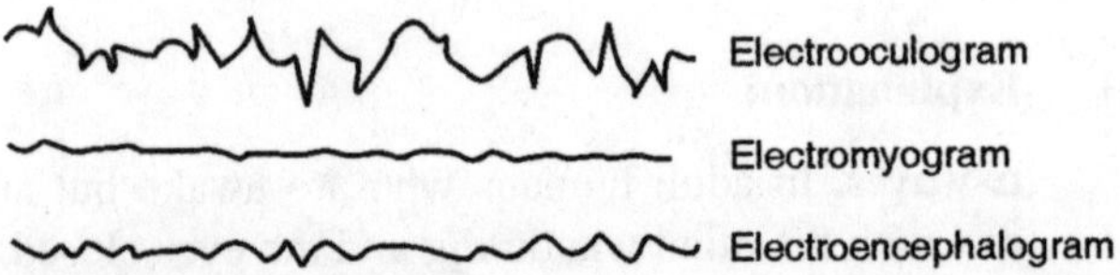

Ans. (C)

Explanation:

In REM sleep: Rapid low voltage EEG activity is seen. Since EEG activity is rapid, so called **paradoxical sleep**.

- Rapid, roving movements of eyes occur → which can be recorded from **EOG (Electro-oculogram)**.
- Occurrence of large phasic potentials in groups of 3-5 that originate in **pons**

↓

Ponto-geniculo-occipital spikes (**PGO**)
- go to
- ↓
- LGB (Lateral geniculate bodies)
- ↓
- Occipital cortex

- Tone of skeletal muscles in neck is markedly reduced also seen in **electromyogram**.

4. High-frequency stimulation of which of the following does not produce the alerting response?

A. Sciatic nerve
B. Lateral spinothalamic tract
C. Midbrain reticular formation
D. Medial lemniscus above the midbrain
E. Intralaminar nuclei of the thalamus

Ans. (D)

Explanation:

High frequency stimulation of the **midbrain reticular formation** produces EEG alerting response and arouses a sleeping animal while stimulation of these systems above midbrain, stimulation of specific sensory relay nuclei of thalamus or stimulation of cortical receiving areas themselves **does not** produce the alerting response.

5. A localized lesion in which of the following structures would be expected to produce prolonged coma?

A. Nucleus tractus solitarius
B. Locus ceruleus
C. Right frontal lobe
D. Both frontal lobe
E. Periaqueductal region at top of midbrain

Ans. (E)

Explanation:

It causes lesion of RAS leading to coma state.

6. Regular rhythmic fluctuations in electrical activity are observed in the cerebral cortex and thalamus. In addition, they are seen in the:

A. Mediobasal portion of the hypothalamus
B. Cerebellar cortex
C. Midbrain reticular formation
D. Amygdala
E. Pons

Ans. (B)

Explanation:

Nuclei concerned with efferent control mechanisms include several nuclei that are concerned with motor function. They receive input from the basal ganglia and the cerebellum and project to the motor cortex. *(Pg. 192)*

7. In which of the following is blood flow *not* increased in REM sleep?

A. Primary visual cortex
B. Anterior cingulate cortex
C. Pons
D. Visual association cortex
E. Amygdalas

Ans. (A)

Explanation:

During REM sleeps, increased activity is seen in **pontine areas, amygdala and cingulate** gyrus but decreased activity in prefrontal and parietal cortex.
Activity in visual association areas is increased, but there is a decrease in activity in primary visual cortex. This is consistent with increased emotion and operation of a closed neural system cut off from the areas that relate brain activity to the external world. *(Pg.199)*

8. Narcolepsy is triggered by abnormalities in:

A. Skeletal muscles
B. Medulla oblongata
C. Hypothalamus
D. Olfactory bulb
E. Neocortex

Ans. (D)

Explanation:

Narcolepsy is a disease characterized by episodic sudden loss of muscle tone and an eventual irresistible urge to sleep during daytime activities. *(Pg. 201)*

9. Frequency of episodes of REM sleep after first falling asleep is:

A. Greater than frequency of episodes of REM sleep after 6 hours of sleep

B. Same as frequency of episodes of REM sleep after 6 hours of sleep

C. Less than frequency of episodes of REM sleep after 6 hours of sleep

Ans. (C)

Explanation:

A young adult first enters NREM sleep, passes through stages 1 & 2 and spends 70-100 minutes in stages 3 & 4. Sleep then lightens and an REM period follows. This cycle is repeated at intervals of about 90 min throughout night. Thus 4-6 REM periods/night. *(Pg. 199)*

10. Percentage of total sleep time spent in REM sleep in neonates is:

A. Greater than percentage of total sleep time spent in REM sleep in adults

B. Same as percentage of total sleep time spent in REM sleep in adults

C. Less than percentage of total sleep time spent in REM sleep in adults

Ans. (A)

Explanation:

REM sleep occupies 80% of total sleep time in premature infants and 50% in full term neonates. Thereafter percentage of REM sleep falls rapidly and plateaus at about 25% until it falls further in old age. *(Pg. 199-200)*

Chapter 12 Control of Posture and Movement

In questions 1-4 refer to Figure below. Structures identified by letter may be selected once, more than once, or not at all.

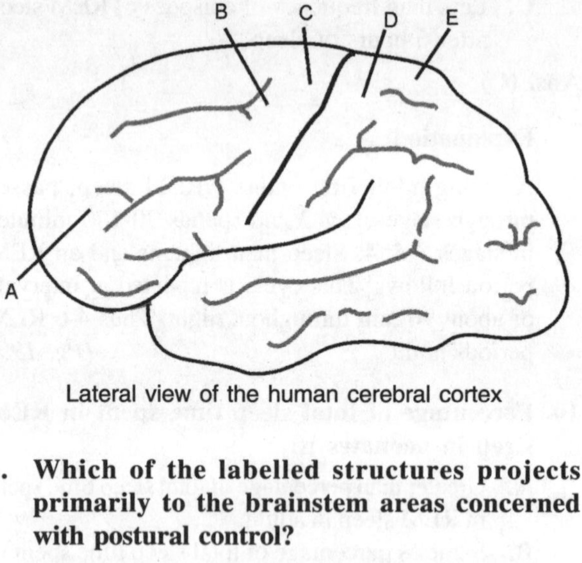

Lateral view of the human cerebral cortex

1. Which of the labelled structures projects primarily to the brainstem areas concerned with postural control?

Ans. (B) Supplementary motor area

(Guyton, 20th Ed., Fig. 55-1, Pg. 686)

2. Which of the labelled structures is concerned with elaboration of somatic sensory perception?

Ans. (E)

Explanation:

Somatic association areas play important roles in deciphering deeper meanings of the sensory information. When somatosensory association area is removed on one side of the brain, the person loses ability to recognize complex objects and complex forms felt on opposite side of body.

This complex sensory deficit is called **amorphosynthesis.**

(Guyton, Pg. 592)

3. Which of the labelled structures is concerned with the primary perception of tactile stimuli?

Ans. (D) Somatosensory area

4. Which of the labeled structures is the supplementary motor area?

Ans. (B)

5. A primary function of the basal ganglia is:

A. Sensory integration
B. Short-term memory
C. Planning voluntary movement
D. Neuroendocrine control
E. Slow-wave sleep

Ans. (C)

Explanation:

Basal ganglia is primarily involved in planning and programming of movement. *(Pg. 214)*

6. The therapeutic effect of L-dopa in patients with Parkinson's disease eventually wears off because:

A. Antibodies to dopamine receptors develop
B. Inhibitory pathways grow into the basal ganglia from the frontal lobe
C. There is an increase in circulating α-synuclein
D. The normal action of NGF is disrupted
E. The dopaminergic neurons in the subtstantia nigra continue to degenerate

Ans. (E)

Explanation:

L-dopa will cross blood brain barrier and helps repair dopamine deficiency in Parkinson's disease.

However, the degeneration of neurons continues and in 5-7 years, the beneficial effects of L-dopa disappear. *(Pg. 217)*

7. Increased neural activity before a skilled voluntary movement is first seen in the:

A. Spinal motor neurons
B. Precentral motor cortex
C. Midbrain
D. Cerebellum
E. Cortical association areas

Ans. (E)

(Pg. 272)

8. After falling down a flight of stairs, a young woman is found to have partial loss of voluntary movement on the right side of her body and loss of pain and temperature sensation on the left side below the midthoracic region. It is probable that she has a lesion:

A. Transecting the left half of the spinal cord in the lumbar region
B. Transecting the left half of the spinal cord in the upper thoracic region
C. Transecting sensory and motor pathways on the right side of the pons
D. Transecting the right half of the spinal cord in the upper thoracic region
E. Transecting the dorsal half of the spinal cord in the upper thoracic region

Ans. (D)

Explanation:

Because of crossing of **lateral spinothalamic tracts** which carry pain and temperature sensation. *(Pg. 139)*

While **corticospinal tract** *(Pg 204)*, 80% of fibers (lateral corticospinal tract) cross the midline in the medullary pyramids only, finally terminating principally on the interneurons in the intermediate regions of the cord grey matter, a few terminate on sensory relay neurons in the dorsal horn and a few terminate directly on anterior motor neurons that cause muscle contraction and are concerned with skilled movements. A few of fibers do not cross to the opposite side in the medulla but pass ipsilaterally down the cord in (ventral) anterior corticospinal tracts (20%). These fibers eventually cross to the opposite side of the cord either in the neck or in the upper thoracic region. These fibers may be concerned with control of bilateral postural movements by the supplementary motor cortex.

(Guyton, 20th Ed, Pg. 687; Ganong, Pg. 204)

9. Patients with transected spinal cords frequently have a negative nitrogen balance because:

A. They develop hypercalcemia, and this causes dissolution of the protein in bone
B. They are paralyzed below the level of the transection
C. They lack the afferent input that normally maintains growth hormone secretion
D. They have difficulty voiding, and this causes nitrogen to accumulate in the urine in the bladder
E. Their ACTH response to stress is reduced

Ans. (B)

Explanation:

Because of immobilization, patients develop negative nitrogen balance and catabolize large amounts of body protein. *(Pg. 208)*

10. Which of the following diseases in not known to be caused by overexpression of a trinucleotide repeat?

A. Alzheimer's disease
B. Fragile X syndrome
C. Spinocerebeller ataxia, type 3
D. Huntington's disease
E. Friedreich's ataxia

Ans. (A)

Explanation:

Alzheimer's disease is due to aggregation of $A\beta_{1-40}$ and $A\beta_{1-42}$ peptides with formation of plaques.

(Pg. 270)

While

Huntington's disease Spinocerebellar ataxia Fragile X syndrome Friedreich's ataxia Myotonic dystrophy	Due to expanded trinucleotide repeat expansion

(Pg. 215)

Chapter 13 The Autonomic Nervous System

1. Complete denervation of the small intestine would be expected to:

A. Cause atrophy of the enteric nervous system
B. Increase the resting rate of intestinal peristalsis
C. Have little effect on the resting rate of intestinal peristalsis
D. Abolish the intestinal response to stretch
E. Cause peristalsis to become chaotic and irregular

Ans. (C)

Explanation:

Peristaltic activity can be increased or decreased by the autonomic input to the gut, but its occurrence is independent of the extrinsic innervation (extrinsic innervation from autonomic nervous system, ANS). *(Pg. 480)*

2. Which of the following drugs would not be expected to increase sympathetic discharge or mimic the effects of increased sympathetic discharge?

A. Prazosin
B. Neostigmine
C. Amphetamine
D Isoproterenol
E. Methoxamine

Ans. (A)

Explanation:

Prazosin is a α_1 blocker:
Rest *(Pg. 230)*

Neostigmine	-	Inhibits acetylcholinesterase	Arguments autonomic activity.
Amphetamine	-	Releases NE	
Isoproterenol	-	Stimulates β receptors	
Methoxamine	-	Stimulates α_1 receptors	

In question 3-8, one or more of the answers may be correct select:

A. If (1), (2) and (3) are correct
B. If (1) and (3) are correct
C. If (2) and (4) are correct
D. If only (4) is correct
E. If all are correct

3. Administration of physostigmine, a drug that inhibits acetylcholinesterase, would be expected to:

1. Increase the secretion of gastric juice
2. Increase the rate of melatonin synthesis and secretion from the pineal gland
3. Increase the rate of epinephrine secretion from the adrenal medulla
4. Decrease the secretion of glucagon

Ans. (A)

Explanation:

- **Physostigmine** inhibits acetylcholinesterase at the site of sympathetic and parasympathetic ganglia therefore augments activity of autonomic nervous system. *(Pg. 230)*
- The cholinergic preganglionic neurons to the adrenal medulla are the secretomotor nerves to the gland.The post ganglionic cells of adrenal medulla have lost their axons and secrete NE, epinephrine and some dopamine directly into the blood stream. *(Pg. 224)*

4. In low doses, nicotine:

1. Acts directly on intestinal smooth muscle, causing it to contract
2. Increases the rate of discharge of postganglionic parasympathetic neurons
3. Decreases the release of acetylcholine in sympathetic ganglia
4. Increases the rate of discharge of postganglionic sympathetic neurons

Ans. (C)

Explanation:

Nicotine stimulates postganglionic neurons of both sympathetic and parasympathetic system because it augments autonomic activity. *(Pg. 230)*

5. In the parasympathetic nervous system:

1. The axons of the preganglionic neurons are in the ventral roots of the spinal nerves in the sacral region
2. The axons of the preganglionic neurons are in the ventral roots of the spinal nerves in the lower thoracic and lumbar regions
3. Dopamine is the neurotransmitter responsible for transmission from preganglionic neurons to postganglionic neurons
4. The axons of postganglionic neurons are usually shorter than those of preganglionic neurons

Ans. (D)

Explanation:

The preganglionic fibers end on short postganglionic neurons located on or near the visceral structures so postganglionic fibers are shorter.

6. Administration of a drug that blocks conversion of L-dopa to dopamine would be expected to:

1. Increase the diameter of the trachea and bronchi
2. Disrupt the function of the SIF cells in the sympathetic ganglia
3. Decrease peristaltic activity in the small intestine
4. Decrease the amount of norepinephrine in the circulating blood

Ans (C)

Explanation:

Small, intensely fluorescent cells (SIF) are the

interneurons that secrete dopamine in the ganglia. Synthesis of catecholamines occurs due to dopamine and if dopamine is deficient, NE and E are not synthesized.

Phenylalanine
↓Phenylalanine hydroxylase
Tyrosine
↓Tyrosine hydroxylase
Dopa (dihydroxy phenylalanine)
↓aminoacid decarboxylase
Dopamine
↓dopamine-β-hydroxylase
Norepinephrine
↓phenylethanolamine-N-methyltransferase (PNMT)
Epinephrine

Both E and NE are metabolized to biologically inactive products by **oxidation** (by MAO monoamine oxidase) and **methylation** (COMT) (Catechol-O-methyl transferase).

(Pg. 103)

7. Administration of a drug that blocks β-adrenergic receptors would be expected to:

1. Decrease the heart rate
2. Decrease the force of cardiac contraction
3. Decrease the secretion of renin from the kidneys
4. Decrease the secretion of insulin from the B cells in the pancreatic islets

Ans. (E)

Explanation:

- Noradrenergic discharge via β receptors accelerates heartbeat and increases contractility.
- Also leads to elevated plasma glucose and FFA levels (supplying more energy).
- Stimulation of the renal nerves increases renin secretion by a direct action of released NE on β_1 adrenergic receptors on the juxtaglomerular cells. So **blockage of β adrenergic receptors** would reverse whole of these effects. *(Pg. 705)*

8. Polypeptides found in the autonomic nervous system include:

1. Gonadotropin-releasing hormone (GnRH)
2. Neuropeptide γ
3. Gastrin-releasing peptide (GRP)
4. Vasoactive intestinal polypeptide (VIP)

Ans. (E)

Explanation:

- GnRH is secreted by some of preganglionic neurons. It mediates a slow excitatory response. In addition there are cotransmitters in ANS e.g.
- VIP is released with acetylcholine. *(Pg. 224)*
- ATP and neuropeptide γ with NE.
- GRP is present in vagal nerve endings that terminate on G cells and is the neurotransmitter producing vagally mediated increases in gastric secretion. *(Pg. 487)*

9. Gastric acid secretion after removal of the celiac ganglion is:

A. Greater than gastric acid secretion after vagotomy
B. Same as gastric acid secretion after vagotomy
C. Less than gastric acid secretion after vagotomy

Ans. (A)

Explanation:

Vagus stimulates gastric acid release while coeliac ganglia being sympathetic ganglia decreases gastric acid secretion, so vagotomy decreases gastric acid secretion.

(Pg. 228)

10. Number of B fibers in white ramus communicans is:

A. Greater than number of B fibers in gray ramus communicans

B. Same as number of B fibers in gray ramus communicans

C. Less than number of B fibers in gray ramus communicans

Ans. (A)

Explanation:

The cell bodies of preganglionic neurons are located in the visceral efferent intermediolateral gray column of spinal cord or the homologus motor nuclei of the cranial nerves. Their axons are mostly myelinated, relatively slow conducting B fibers.

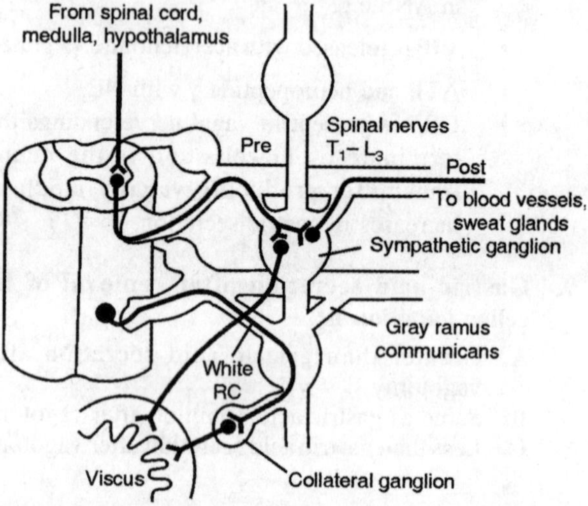

Diagram showing sympathetic division of ANS

UNIT III. NERVOUS SYSTEM

Chapter 14 Central Regulation of Visceral Function

1. Thirst is stimulated by:

- **A.** Increases in plasma osmolality and volume
- **B.** An increase in plasma osmolality and a decrease in plasma volume
- **C.** A decrease in plasma osmolality and an increase in plasma volume
- **D.** Decreases in plasma osmolality and volume
- **E.** Injection of vasopressin into the hypothalamus

Ans. (C)

Explanation:

- Drinking is regulated by plasma osmolality and ECF volume. Water intake is increased by effective osmotic pressure of the plasma and decreases in ECF volume and by psychologic and other factors.
- **Osmolality acts via** osmoreceptors (receptors that sense the osmolality of body fluids). These osmoreceptors are located in the anterior hypothalamus.
- **Decreases in ECF volume also** stimulate thirst by a pathway independent of that mediating thirst in response to increased plasma osmolality. Effect of ECF volume depletion on thirst is mediated in part via the renin-angiotensin system.

Hypertonicity
↓
Osmoreceptors
(Ant. hypothalamus **OVLT**)

Hypovolemia
↓
Baroreceptors
Angiotensin II
(Subfornical organ)

THIRST
Hypothalamus (Lateral superior)
(Integrating area)

Angiotension II acts on subfornical organ (SFO) and possibly on the OVLT (Organum vasculosum of the lamina terminalis) to increase water intake. In addition it appears that OVLT is the site of the osmoreceptor controlling vasopressin secretion.

(Pg. 240-241)

2. A gain-of-function mutation in which of the following genes would be expected to cause obesity in humans?

A. Leptin
B. Leptin receptor
C. Thyrotropin β subunit
D. Pro-opiomelanocortin
E. Melanin-concentrating hormone

Ans. (E)

Explanation:

Polypeptide that increases food intake in mammals is melanin-concentrating hormone (MCH), a polypeptide which is secreted by the pituitary in fish. In mammals, found only in lateral hypothalamus, while pro-opiomelanocortion (POMC) derivatives, particularly α-MSH decrease food intake. Also leptin and its receptors inhibit food intake. *(Pg. 238)*

3. When an individual is naked in a room in which the air temperature is 21°C (69.8°C) and the humidity 80%, the greatest amount of heat is lost from the body by:

A. Elevated metabolism
B. Respiration
C. Urination
D. Vaporization of sweat
E. Radiation and conduction

Ans. (E)

Explanation:

- **Radiation** is loss of heat in the form of infrared heat waves (**electromagnetic wave)** while in **Conduction** heat exchange occurs from the surface of one object to the surface of another and is aided by convection.

(Guyton, 20th Ed., Pg. 891)

- Percentage of heat lost at 21°C is 60-70% by conduction and radiation.

4. Secretion of which of the following hormones does *not* increase at night?

A. Growth hormone
B. ACTH
C. Melatonin
D. Insulin
E. Prolactin

Ans. (D)

Explanation:

Most of the cells in the body have circadian rhythms. These rhythms are entrained (i.e. synchronized to a day-light cycle) by the paired suprachiasmatic nuclei (SCN), one on either side, above the optic chiasma. These nuclei receive information about the light-dark cycle via a special neural pathway, the **retinohypothalamic fibers** that pass from the optic chiasma to the SCN. Efferent from SCN initiate neural and humoral signals that entrain a wide variety of well known circadian rhythms. These include rhythms in the secretion of **ACTH** and **other pituitary hormones**, the sleep-wake cycle, the body temperature cycle, and the secretion of the pineal hormone **melatonin**. *(Pg. 235)*

Questions 5-10 refer to figure below. Each lettered structure may be selected once, more than once, or not at all.

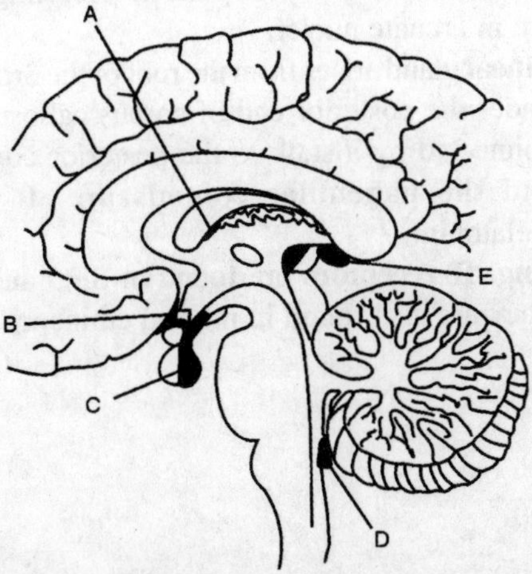

5. **Which of the labeled structures has the highest concentration of angiotensin II receptors?**
   Ans. (A)
6. **Which of the labeled structures has the highest concentration of corticotropin-releasing hormone (CRH)?**
   Ans. (C)
7. **Which of the labeled structures has the highest concentration of thyrotropin-releasing hormone (TRH)?**
   Ans. (C)
8. **Which of the labeled structures has the highest concentration of dopamine?**
   Ans. (E)
9. **Which of the labeled structures has the highest concentration of growth hormone-releasing hormone (GRH)?**
   Ans. (E)
10. **Which of the labeled structures is most involved in the regulation of circadian rhythms?**
    Ans. (B)

Explanation:

- **GnRH** secreting neurons are primarily in the medial preoptic areas. *(Pg. 249)*
- **Somatostatin** secreting neurons are in the paraventricular nuclei.
- **GRH** secreting and **dopamine** secreting neurons are in arcuate nuclei.
- **Pineal** gland arises from the roof of the 3rd ventricle under the posterior end of corpus callosum and is connected by a stalk to the posterior commissure and the habenular commissure. It secretes melatonin. *(Pg. 462)*
- **Ang. II receptors** are found in SFO and OVLT. They are also found in median eminence. *(Pg. 250)*

Chapter 15 Neural Basis of Instinctual Behavior and Emotions

Questions 1-6 are made up of a statement and an explanation. Select:

A. If both the statement and the explanation are true and they are related

B. If both the statement and explanation are true but they are unrelated

C. If the statement is true but the explanation is false

D. If the statement is false but the explanation is true, and

E. If the statement and the explanation are both false

1. L-Dopa is of benefit in the treatment of Parkinson's disease because it increases the dopamine content of the tuberoinfundibular dopaminergic neurons.

Ans. (B)

Explanation:

The brain has many dopaminergic systems. Tuberoinfundibular system is that which secretes the dopamine into the portal hypophysial vessels and inhibit prolactin secretion. In **Parkinson's disease, there is degeneration of nigrostriatal dopaminergic neurons**. The nigrostriatal system, projects from the substantia nigra to the striatum and is involved in motor control. L-dopa crosses bloodbrain barrier (BBB) and helps repair dopamine deficiency.

(Pg. 216, 263)

2. Drugs that decrease serotonin reuptake are of benefit in the treatment of some depressive illnesses because they increase extracellular norepinephrine in the brain.

Ans. (C)

Explanation:

In patients who are depressed, the primary serotonin metabolite (5-HIAA) is low in CSF. It used to be argued that depression is caused by low extracellular NE (norepinephrine) in the brain and drugs that inhibit NE reuptake were of considerable value in the treatment of depression. However these drugs also inhibit serotonin reuptake, e.g., Prozac, fluoxetine, which inhibit serotonin reuptake without affecting NE reuptake, are equally effective as antidepressants. So the focus in treating clinical depression has shifted from NE to serotonin.

(Pg. 263)

3. Procedures that increase the release of opioid peptides in the central nervous system decrease the effect of painful stimuli because the peptides bind to μ receptors.

Ans. (A)

Explanation:

There are at least 3 nonmutually exclusive sites at which opiods could act to produce analgesia.

- Periphery.
- At the site of an injury.
- In dorsal horn where nociceptive fibers synapse on the dorsal root ganglion cells.
- At more rostral sites in the brainstem.

The opoid receptors (μ) in the dorsal horn region could act presynaptically to decrease release of **substance P.** *(Pg. 146)*

4. The antipsychotic activity of the major tranquilizers parallels their ability to block serotonin receptors because the serotonergic neural system in the brain are concerned, among other things, with normal mental function.

Ans. (B)

Explanation:

- **Tranquilizers** are the drugs that allay anxiety and various psychiatric symptoms. *(Pg. 261)*
- The increase in Cl^- conductance produced by $GABA_A$ receptors is potentiated by the benzodiazepines, drugs that have marked antianxiety activity and are also effective muscle relaxants. *(Pg. 110)*
- Serotonin is important as antidepressant. *(See Q. 2)*

5. Women with a congenital adrenocortical enzyme defect that cause large amounts of androgens to be secreted have somewhat more masculine behavior than normal woman because the androgens act on the brain during fetal development.

Ans. (A)

Explanation:

The characteristic pattern that develops in females in the absence of treatment is the **adrenogenital syndrome.** Musculization may not be marked until later in life and mild cases can be detected only by laboratory tests. *(Pg. 366)*

6. Increased anxiety is produced by $GABA_B$ receptors, so treatment with $GABA_B$ antagonists has an antianxiety effect:

Ans. (B) *(Pg. 259)*

Explanation:

- Tranquilizers are the drugs that allay anxiety and various psychiatric symptoms. *(Pg. 261)*
- The increase in Cl^- conductance produced by $GABA_A$ receptors is potentiated by the benzodiazepines, drugs that have marked anti-

anxiety activity and are also effective muscle relaxants. *(Pg. 110)*

- Serotonin is important as antidepressant. *(See Q. 2)*

7. Which of the following would be expected to reduce maternal behavior?

A. Lesions of the occipital cortex
B. Lesions of the mediobasal hypothalamus
C. Loss of expression of the gene for Fos-B
D. Ovariectomy
E. Hysterectomy

Ans. (C)

Explanation:

Knock out of the Fos-B gene, one of the family of early fos genes is associated with failure to retrieve and care for pups after delivery in female mice. *(Pg. 259)*

8. The cell bodies of the principal histaminergic neurons in the brain are located in the:

A. Preoptic area of the hypothalamus
B. Central nucleus of the amygdala
C. Subfornical organ
D. Locus ceruleus
E. Mediobasal hypothalamus

Ans. (E)

Explanation:

Histaminergic neurons have their cell bodies in the tuberomamillary nucleus in the ventral portion of the posterior hypothalamus. The axons of these neurons project to all parts of the brain. Evidence links brain histamine to arousal, sexual behavior, blood pressure, drinking, pain thresholds and regulation of secretion of several anterior pituitary hormones. *(Pg. 264)*

9. Which of the following drugs is a tranquilizer?

A. LSD
B. Atropine
C. Ecstasy (MDMA)
D. Lithium
E. Chlorpromazine

Ans. (E)

Explanation:

- **Hallucinogenic** agent **lysergic acid diethylamide** (LSD) is a serotonin agonist that produces its effects by activating 5-HT_2 receptors in the brain.
- Ecstasy (MDMD or 3,4-Methylene dioxy-methamphetamine) is a drug of abuse because of its hallucinogenic properties. The drug produces euphoria because of release of serotonin. *(Pg. 262)*
- Lithium is used as antidepressant.

10. In which of the following diseases is there reason to believe that the mesocortical system of dopaminergic neurons is hyperactive?

A. Parkinson's disease
B. Bipolar disorder
C. Schizophrenia
D. Hyperprolactinemia
E. Migraine

Ans. (C)

Explanation:

A large amount of evidence suggests that defect in mesocortical system (i.e. system that projects to nucleus accumbens and is involved in reward behavior and addiction). It also projects to related limbic subcortical areas and is responsible for development of at least some of the symptoms of schizophrenia. However, amphetamine like drugs which causes release of dopamine as well as NE in brain causes schizophrenia like psychosis. Brain levels of D_2 receptors are said to be elevated in schizophrenia and there is clear positive correlation between the antischizophrenic activity of many drugs and their ability to block D_2 receptors.

(Pg. 263-264)

11. Perception of disgust appears to depend on the:

A. Frontal cortex
B. Postcentral gyrus on the right side
C. Postcentral gyrus on the left side
D. Insular cortex on the right side
E. Insular cortex on the left side

Ans. (E)

Explanation:

Patient with selective lesions of left insula and putamen experienced difficulty recognizing disgust on the faces or in the voices of people the patient met. *(Pg. 260)*

12. Area of brain where animals will avoid stimulation through an implanted electrode is:

A. Greater than the area of brain where animals will work to receive repeated stimulation through an implanted electrode
B. Same as the area of brain where animals will work to receive repeated stimulation through an implanted electrode
C. Less than the area of brain where animals will work to receive repeated stimulation through an implanted electrode

Ans. (C)

Explanation:

The **areas in the brain where stimulation leads to repeated bar pressing** are:

- Ventral segmentum.
- Medial forebrain bundle.
- Nucleus accumbens.
- Frontal cortex.

The **most responsive area** is the **dopaminergic** pathway from ventral segmental area to the **nucleus accumbens.**

The points where stimulation is avoided are in:

- Lateral portion of posterior hypothalamus.
- Dorsal midbrain.
- Entorhinal cortex.

The areas where bar **pressing** is **repeated** are much **more** extensive than those where it is **avoided**. It has been calculated that in rats **repeated pressing** is obtained from **35%** of the brain, avoidance from 5%.

- Indifferent response–from 60%. *(Pg. 260)*

13. Amount of norepinephrine in the raphe nuclei:

A. Greater than the amount of serotonin in the raphe nuclei

B. Same as the amount of serotonin in the raphe nuclei

C. Less than the amount of serotonin in the raphe nuclei

Ans. (C)

Explanation:

- Serotonin containing neurons have their cell bodies in the midline raphe nuclei of the brainstem and project to portions of hypothalamus, the limbic system, the neocortex, cerebellum and the spinal cord. *(Pg. 262)*
- The cell bodies of the NE containing neurons in the brain are located in locus ceruleus and the nuclei in the pons and medulla. From the locus ceruleus, the axons of the noradrenergic neurons form the **locus ceruleus system.** *(Pg. 263)*

UNIT III. NERVOUS SYSTEM

Chapter 16 Higher Functions of the Nervous System

1. **Retrograde amnesia:**
   - **A.** Is abolished by prefrontal lobotomy
   - **B.** Responds to drugs that block dopamine receptors
   - **C.** Is commonly precipitated by a blow on the head
   - **D.** Is increased by administration of vasopressin
   - **E.** Is due to damage to the brainstem

Ans: (C)

Explanation:

Retrograde amnesia means loss of memory for the events immediately preceding brain concussion/electroshock therapy. This amnesia encompasses longer periods than it does in experimental animals–sometimes many days–but remote memories remain intact. *(Pg. 269)*

2. **The representational hemisphere:**
   - **A.** Is the right cerebral hemisphere in most right-handed individuals
   - **B.** Is the left cerebral hemisphere in most left-handed individuals
   - **C.** Includes the part of the brain concerned with language functions
   - **D.** Is the site of lesions in most patients with aphasia
   - **E.** Is morphologically identical to the opposite nonrepresentational hemisphere

Ans: (A)

Explanation:

Dominant (categorical hemisphere) is concerned with sequential-analytic process (**language**

function) while **representational** hemisphere is concerned with **visuospatial** relations (i.e. identification of objects by their form and the recognition of musical themes). It is also concerned with recognition of faces. Hemispheric specialization (91% of people) is related to handedness. In 96% of right handed people, left hemisphere is the categorical hemisphere, while right hemisphere is the representational hemisphere. *(Pg. 273)*

3. The optic chiasm and corpus callosum are sectioned in a dog, and with the right eye covered, the animal is trained to bark when it sees a red square. The right eye is then uncovered and the left eye covered. The animal will now:

A. Fail to respond to the red square because the square does not produce impulses that reach the right occipital cortex
B. Fail to respond to the red square because the animal has bitemporal hemianopia
C. Fail to respond to the red square if the posterior commissure is also sectioned
D. Respond to the red square only after retraining
E. Respond promptly to the red square in spite of the lack of input to the left occipital cortex

Ans. **(E)**

Explanation:

Memory transfer occurs in the anterior portion of the corpus callosum. Neural coding for remembering with one eye what has been learned with the other will be transferred to the opposite cortex via the commissures. *(Pg. 268)*

4. The effects of bilateral loss of hippocampal function include:

A. Disappearance of remote memories
B. Loss of the ability to encode events of the recent past in long-term memory

C. Loss of ability to recall faces and forms but not the ability to recall printed or spoken words
D. Loss of the ability to recall faces and forms but not the ability to recall printed or spoken words
E. Production of inappropriate emotional responses when recalling events of the recent past

Ans. (C)

Explanation:

Bilateral destruction of ventral hippocampus/ Alzheimer's disease or similar disease that destroys CA1 neurons, cause striking defects in short term memory. Humans with such destruction have intact working memory and remote memory. They are capable of new learning and retain old prelesion memories, but they cannot form new long-term memories. *(Pg. 269)*

5. **Which of the following are *incorrectly* paired?**
   A. Lesion of the parietal lobe of the representational hemisphere: unilateral inattention and neglect
   B. Loss of cholinergic neurons in the nucleus basalis of Meynert and related areas of the forebrain: loss of recent memory
   C. Lesions of mamillary bodies: loss of recent memory
   D. Lesion of the angular gyrus in the categorical hemisphere: nonfluent aphasia
   E. Lesion of Broca's area in the categorical hemisphere: slow speech

Ans: (D)

Explanation:

When a lesion damages the angular gyrus in the categorical hemisphere without affecting the Wernicke's or Broca's areas, there is no difficulty with speech or the understanding of auditory information, instead there is trouble understanding written language or pictures, because visual information is not processed and transmitted to Wernicke's area. This condition is called **anomic aphasia**. *(Pg. 275)*

Other aphasias	**Site of lesion**
Non-fluent aphasia	Broca's area
Fluent aphasia	Wernicke's area
Conduction aphasia	Lesions of arcuate fasciculus connecting Wernicke's and Broca's areas

The angular gyrus behind Wernicke's area appears to process information from words that are read in such a way that they can be converted into the auditory forms of the words in Wernicke's area. *(Pg. 274)*

6. The representational hemisphere is better than the categorical hemisphere at:

A. Language functions
B. Recognition of objects by their form
C. Understanding printed words
D. Understanding spoken words
E. Mathematical calculations

Ans. (B)

Explanation:

Dominant (categorical hemisphere) is concerned with sequential-analytic process (**language function**) while **representational** hemisphere is concerned with **visuospatial** relations (i.e. identification of objects by their form and the recognition of musical themes). It is also concerned with recognition of faces. Hemispheric specialization is related to handedness. In 96% of right (91% of people) handed people, left hemisphere is the categorical hemisphere, while right hemisphere is the representational hemisphere. *(Fig. 16.6, Pg. 273)*

7. Which of the following in *not* characteristic of conditioned reflexes?

A. Failure to form conditioned reflexes when the conditioned and unconditioned stimuli are separated by more than 2 minutes

B. Disappearance of the conditioned reflex if it is not reinforced from time to time

C. Rapid formation of conditioned reflexes when the conditioned stimulus is pleasant for the animal

D. Failure to form of conditioned reflexes when the conditioned stimulus is unpleasant to the animal

E. Failure to form conditioned reflexes when, after the conditioned stimulus, there is a distracting stimulus before the unconditioned stimulus

Ans. (D)

Explanation:

If the animal is disturbed by an external stimulus immediately after the **CS (conditioned stimulus)** is applied, the conditioned response may not occur (**external inhibition**). Conditioned reflexes are difficult to form unless the **US (unconditional stimulus)** is associated with a pleasant or unpleasant effect. Stimulation of the brain reward system is a powerful **US (positive reinforcement)** or so is stimulation of the avoidance system or a painful shock to the skin (**negative reinforcement).**

(Pg. 268)

8. A lesion of Wernicke's area (the posterior end of the superior temporal gyrus) in the categorical hemisphere causes patients to:

A. Lose short-term memory

B. Speak in slow, halting voice

C. Experience déjá vu

D. Talk rapidly but make little sense

E. Lose the ability to recognize faces

Ans. (D)

Explanation:

In Wernicke's area lesion, speech itself is normal and sometimes patients talk excessively, but it is full of jargon and neologisms that make little sense. Patient also fails to comprehend the meaning of spoken or written words. Wernicke's area is concerned with comprehension of auditory and visual information. *(Pg. 273-274)*

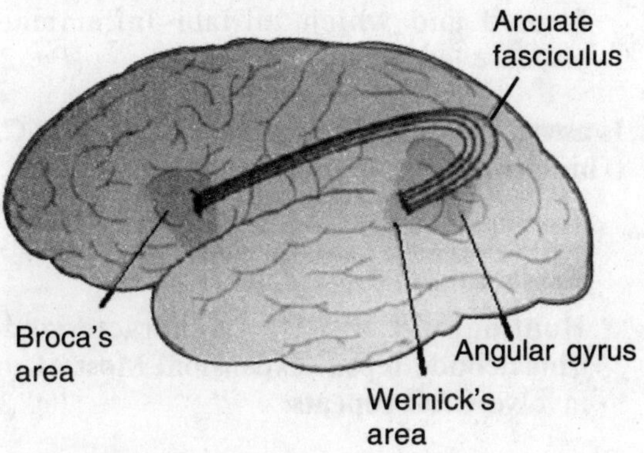

Location of some of the areas in the categorical hemisphere that are concerned with language development.

Q. In the following select:

A. If the item is associated with (a) below
B. If the item is associated with (b) below
C. If the item is associated with both (a) and (b)
D. If the item is associated with neither (a) nor (b)
(a) Alzheimer's disease
(b) Huntington's disease

9. Affects basal ganglia.

Ans. (B)

Explanation:

Huntington's disease is autosomal dominant disorder affecting basal ganglia

10. Is affected by drugs that inhibit γ-secretase

Ans. (A)

Explanation:

β-amyloid peptides are products of a normal (**senile plaques**) protein, **amyloid precursor protein (APP).** This protein is hydrolyzed at 3 different sites by α, β and γ-secretases respectively. When APP is hydrolyzed by α secretase, non-toxic peptide products are formed, but when it is hydrolyzed by β and γ secretase, toxic polypeptides ($A\beta_{61\text{-}42}$) are formed and which initiate–inflammatory response leading to cell death. *(Pg. 271)*

11. Is associated with an increased number of CAG trinucleotide repeats:

Ans. (B)

Explanation:

Huntington's disease is characterized by trinucleotide repeat expansion. Most of these involve **CAG repeats.** *(Pg. 215)*

12. Affects β-amyloid protein:

Ans. (A)

Explanation:

Cytopathologic hallmarks of Alzheimer's disease are intracellular **neurofibrillary tangles** and extracellular **senile plaques**, which have a core of **β-amyloid peptides.** *(Pg. 271)*

13. Can be cured if treatment is started early in the disease:

Ans. (D)

Explanation:

- Alzheimer's disease is characterized by progressive loss of short-term memory followed by general loss of cognitive and other brain functions.
- Huntington's disease is an autosomal dominant disorder.

Chapter 17 Energy Balance, Metabolism and Nutrition

1. In the body, metabolism of 10 g of protein would produce approximately:

A. 1 kcal
B. 41 kcal
C. 410 kcal
D. 4100 kcal
E. 41 cal

Ans. (B)

Explanation:

Caloric values of the common foodstuffs as measured in a bomb calorimeter are found to be 5.3 kcal/g of protein. In the body, similar values are obtained for carbohydrate and fat but the oxidation of protein is incomplete, the end products of protein catabolism being urea and related nitrogenous compounds in addition to CO_2 and H_2O. Therefore caloric value of **protein** in the body is only **4.1 kcal/kg.** *(Pg. 280)*

2. A man with a respiratory quotient (RQ) of 0.70:

A. Has been eating a high-fat diet
B. Has been eating a high-protein diet
C. Has been fasting for 24 hours
D. Has eaten nothing but carbohydrates for 24 hours
E. Is dehydrated

Ans. (A)

Explanation:

$$\text{Respiratory quotient (RQ)} = \frac{\text{Volume of } CO_2 \text{ produced}}{\text{Volume of } O_2 \text{ consumed}}$$

RQ for carbohydrate = 1
RQ for fat = 0.70
RQ in fat=0.70 because H and O are present in

carbohydrate in the same proportions as in water, whereas in various fats, extra O_2 is necessary for the formation of H_2O.

e.g. **carbohydrate**

$C_6 H_{12} O_6 + 6 O_2 \rightarrow 6 CO_2 + 6H_2O$

RQ= 6/6=1

Fat: $2 C_{15} H_{98}O_6 + 145 O_2 \rightarrow 102 CO_2 + 98H_2O$

RQ= 102/145 = 0.703

(Pg. 280)

3. Which of the following daily intakes (in grams) of carbohydrates (C), protein (P), and fat (F) would be best for a healthy 80 kg male construction worker?

A. C: 420; P: 80; F: 125
B. C: 420; P: 130; F: 100
C. C: 325; P: 80; F: 65
D. C: 550; P: 80; F: 65
E. C: 340; P: 50; F: 65

Ans. (D)

Explanation:

Carbohydrate is the cheapest source of calories and provides 50% or more of the calories in most diets. When calculating dietary needs, it is usual to meet the protein requirement first and then split the remaining calories between fat and carbohydrate, depending on taste, income and other factors, e.g., an 80 kg man who is moderately active needs about 2900 kcal/day.

- Adults should take about 1g/kg body weight protein per day i.e. 80 kg person should take 80 g protein per day. 80 g protein has an energy value of 320 kcal (proteins yield 4 kcal/g and 15% of our calories should come from proteins).
- Total dietary fat should provide less than 30% of the energy intake (1gm of fat provides 9 kcal/g).

- Carbohydrates provide 4 kcal/g and 50% of calories come from carbohydrates. *(Pg. 311)*

4. The major lipoprotein source of the cholesterol used in cells is:

A. Chylomicrons
B. Intermediate-density lipoproteins (IDL)
C. Adbumin-bound free fatty acids
D. LDL
E. HDL

Ans. (D)

Explanation:

LDL provides cholesterol to the tissues. Cholesterol is an essential constituent of cell membranes and is used by gland cells to make steroid hormones. *(Pg. 303)*

5. Which of the following produces the most high-energy phosphate compounds?

A. Aerobic metabolism of 1 mol of glucose
B. Anaerobic metabolism of 1 mol of glucose
C. Metabolism of 1 mol of galactose
D. Metabolism of 1 mol of amino acid
E. Metabolism of 1 mol long-chain fatty acid

Ans. (E)

Explanation:

Catabolism of 1 mol of a six-carbon **fatty acid** through citric acid cycle (CAC) to CO_2 and H_2O leads to:

→ **FA** TCA CO_2 and H_2O
1 mol ⟶ ↓
44 mol of ATP whereas

→ **Glucose** CAC CO_2 and H_2O
1 mol ⟶ ↓
38 mol of ATP *(Pg. 289)*

6. P_{450} (CYP) are found in many parts of the body. In which of the following do they not play an important role?

A. Bile acid formation
B. Carcinogenesis
C. Steroid hormones formation
D. Detoxification of drugs
E. Glycogen synthesis

Ans. (E)

Explanation:

P_{450} also known as CYP (Cytochrome P_{450}) mono oxygenases. The human genome codes 57 of these proteins. They are involved in:

- Eicosanoid synthesis.
- Steroid synthesis.
- Metabolism of FA, fat soluble vitamins.
- Metabolism of carcinogens, and
- Metabolism of many drugs. *(Pg. 310)*

7. Which of the following would not produce an increase in the plasma level of free fatty acids?

A. A drug that increases the level of intracellular cAMP
B. A drug that activates β_3-adrenergic receptors
C. A drug that inhibits hormone-sensitive lipase
D. A drug that decreases the metabolic clearance of glucagon
E. A drug that inhibits phosphodisterase

Ans. (C)

Explanation:

Supply of FFA to the tissues is regulated by 2 lipases.

1. **Lipo-protein lipase** on the surface of the endothelium of the capillaries hydrolyzes the TG's(Triglycerides) in *chylomicrons* and *VLDL*.

$$\text{TG's} \xrightarrow[\text{lipoprotein lipase}]{} \text{FFA} + \text{glycerol} \rightarrow$$

2. **Hormone sensitive lipase** of adipose tissue.

Stored TG's ⟶ FFA + glycerol

Hormone sensitive lipase is converted from inactive to active form by cAMP via protein kinase A.

Catecholamines
↓ via
β_3 receptor
↓
Adenylyl Cyclase (adipose tissue)
ATP ⟶ cAMP
↓
Protein kinase A
↓
Active lipase ← Inactive lipase
↓
TG's → FFA+ glycerol

Adenylyl cyclase is activated by catecholamines

(Pg. 305)

8. When LDL enters cells by receptor-mediated endocytosis, which of the following does not occur?

A. Decrease in the formation of cholesterol from mevalonic acid
B. Increase in the intracellular concentration of cholesteryl eaters
C. Increase in the transfer of cholesterol from the cell to HDL
D. Decreases in the rate of synthesis of LDL receptors
E. Decrease in the cholesterol in endosomes

Ans. (E)

Explanation:

LDL is taken up by receptor-mediated endocytosis in coated pits. The cholesteryl esters enters lysosomes, free cholesterol is released. Cholesterol also:

1. **Inhibits HMG-CoA reductase,** enzyme that converts 3-hydroxy 3-methyl glutaryl coenzyme A (HMG-CoA) to mevalonic acid and form later cholesterol therefore it inhibits its own synthesis.

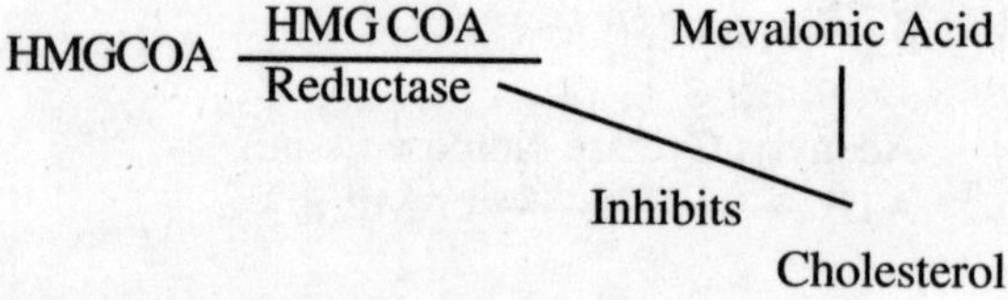

2. Is then processed in part to other cholesteryl esters by the enzyme acetyl CoA.
3. Inhibits formation of LDL receptors.

(Pg. 305)

9. Which of the following does not increase the output of glucose from the liver?

A. Induction of phosphorylase
B. Insulin
C. Glucagon
D. PGC-1
E. Epinephrine

Ans. (B)

Explanation:

Liver takes up glucose from blood stream and stores it as glycogen, but because it also contains glucose 6-phosphatase, it discharges glucose into blood stream. But insulin facilitates glycogen synthesis and inhibits hepatic glucose output. Glycogen contributes to hyperglycaemia and glucose output by the liver is facilitated by catecholamines, cortisol and growth hormone when the stress of illness is severe.

(Pg. 340-341)

10. Spine bifida is associated with deficiency of:

A. Folic acid
B. Vit C
C. Vit B_1
D. Vit K
E. Uric acid

Ans. (A)

Explanation:

Deficiency of folic acid (source of folic acid is from green leafy vegetables) in pregnant female leads to **neural tube** defects in children.

(Pg. 315)

UNIT IV. ENDOCRINOLOGY, METABOLISM AND REPRODUCTIVE FUNCTION

Chapter 18 The Thyroid Gland

1. In which of the following conditions is it most likely that the TSH response to TRH will be reduced?

A. Hypothyroidism due to tissue resistance to thyroid hormone
B. Hypothyroidism due to disease destroying the thyroid gland
C. Hyperthyroidism due to circulating antithyroid antibodies with TSH activity
D. Hyperthyroidism due to diffuse hyperplasia of thyrotropes of the anterior pituitary
E. Iodine deficiency

Ans. (C)

Explanation:

Hyperthyroidism like (Grave's disease) in which antibodies to the TSH receptor stimulate the receptor. This produces marked T_3 and T_4 secretion and enlargement of thyroid gland. However due to *feedback* effects of T_3 and T_4, plasma *TSH* is low. *(Pg. 329)*

2. Methimazole causes:

A. A decrease in thyroid size and an increase in plasma T_4
B. A decrease in both thyroid size and plasma T_4
C. An increase in thyroid size and a decrease in plasma T_4
D. An increase in thyroid size and a decrease in plasma T_4
E. No change in thyroid size and a decrease in plasma T_4

Ans. (D) *(Guyton, Pg. 939)*

Explanation:

- Absence of thyroxine and T_3 in the thyroglobin can lead to tremendous feedback enhancement of TSH secretion by ant. pituitary gland, thus promoting growth of glandular tissue and forming a goiter. *(Pg. 330)*

3. A young woman has puffy skin and a hoarse voice. Her plasma TSH concentration is low but increases markedly when is given TRH. She probably has:

A. Hypothyroidism due to a thyroid tumor
B. Hypothyroidism due to a primary abnormality in the thyroid gland
C. Hypothyroidism due to a primary abnormality in the pituitary gland
D. Hypothyroidism due to a primary abnormality in the hypothalamus
E. Hypothyroidism due to a primary abnormality in the hypothalamus

Ans. (D)

Explanation:

Feedback control by hypothalamus is necessary for maintenance of TSH.

4. The coupling of monoiodotyrosine and diidotyrosine and the iodination of thyroglobulin is blocked by:

A. Divalent cations
B. Monovalent anions such as perchlorate
C. TSH
D. TRH
E. Thiourylenes such as methimazole

Ans. (E)

Explanation:

- **Thiourylenes** are a group of compounds related to thiourea, inhibit the iodination of monoiodotyrosine and block the coupling reaction. Iodination of tyrosine is inhibited because propylthiouracil and methimazole (the 2 used clinically) compete with tyrosine residues for iodine and become iodinated therefore prevents formation of thyroid hormones from iodides and tyrosine.

5. The enzyme primarily responsible for the conversion of T_4 to T_3 in the periphery is:

A. D_1 thyroid deiodinase
B. D_2 thyroid deiodinase
C. D_3 thyroid deiodinase
D. Thyroid peroridase
E. None of the above

Ans. (A)

Explanation:

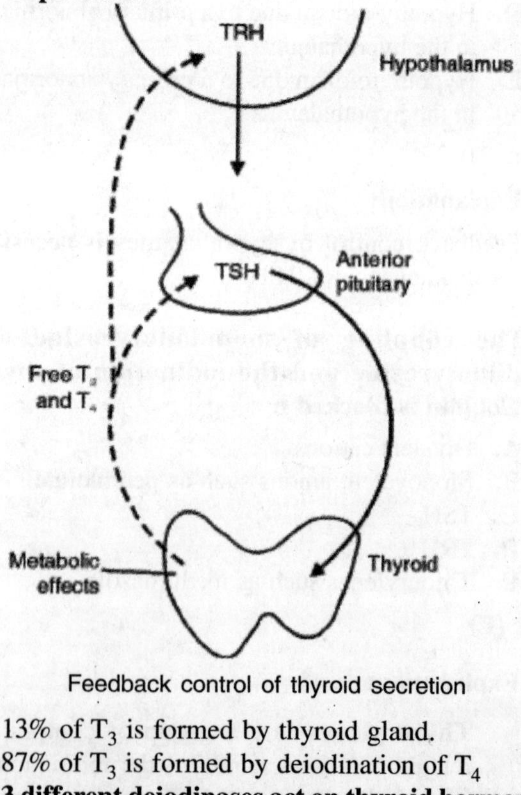

Feedback control of thyroid secretion

13% of T_3 is formed by thyroid gland.
87% of T_3 is formed by deiodination of T_4
3 different deiodinases act on thyroid hormones.

1. D_1
   - Present in liver, kidneys, thyroid and pituitary.
   - Responsible for monitoring the formation of T_3 from T_4 in the periphery.
2. D_2
   - Present in brain, pituitary and brain fat.
   - Also contributes to T_3 formation.
3. D_3
   - Present in brain and in reproductive tissues.
   - Main source of RT_3 in the blood and tissues.

So **deiodinases** appear to be responsible for maintaining the differences in T_3/T_4 ratios in various tissues in the body.

6. The metabolic rate is least affected by an increase in the plasma level of:

A. TSH
B. TRH
C. TBG
D. Free T_4
E. Free T_3

Ans. (C)

Explanation:

Large amounts of T_4 and T_3 are bound to plasma protein e.g. by:
1. Albumin.
2. Thyroxine binding globulin (TBG).
3. Thyroxine binding prealbumin (TBPA, transthyrotin).

- The free thyroid hormones in the plasma are in equilibrium with the protein bound thyroid hormones in plasma and tissues. **It is the free thyroid hormones in plasma that are physiologically active and that inhibit pituitary secretion of TSH.**
- **Function of protein binding**: Appears to be maintenance of a large pool of readily available free hormones. *(Pg. 321)*

7. Which of the following is *not* essential for normal biosynthesis of thyroid hormones?

A. Iodine
B. Ferritin
C. Thyroglobulin
D. Protein synthesis
E. TSH

Ans. (B)

Explanation:

Biosynthesis of thyroid hormones.

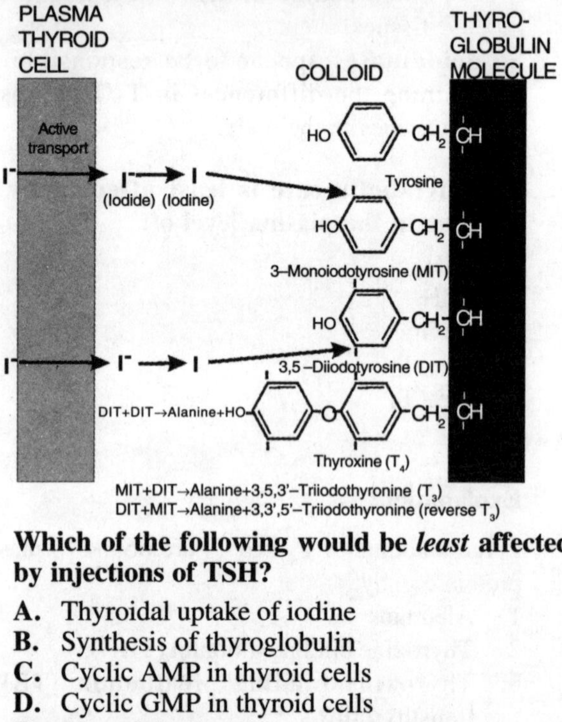

8. Which of the following would be *least* affected by injections of TSH?

A. Thyroidal uptake of iodine
B. Synthesis of thyroglobulin
C. Cyclic AMP in thyroid cells
D. Cyclic GMP in thyroid cells
E. Size of the thyroid

Ans. (D)

Explanation:

- TSH also known as thyrotropin, its specific actions on thyroid gland are as follows:
  1. Increased proteolysis of the thyroglobulin.
  2. Increased activity of the iodine pump.
  3. Increased iodination of tyrosine to form thyroid hormones.

4. Increased size and increased secretory activity of thyroid cells.
5. Increased number of thyroid cells.

- **Mode action:** Via cAMP activation.

Binding of TSH with TSH receptors on cell membrane of thyroid cells
↓
Activation of adenylyl cyclase in membrane
↓
Increases formation of cAMP inside cells
↓
Activation of protein kinase
↓
Phosphorylation inside cell
↓
Increased secretion of **thyroid hormones and growth of thyroid** glandular tissue.

(Guyton, Pg. 938)

9. Hypothyroidism due to disease of the thyroid gland is associated with increased plasma levels of:

A. Cholesterol
B. Albumin
C. RT_3
D. Iodide
E. TBG

Ans. (A)

Explanation:

Thyroid hormones lower circulating cholesterol levels. Therefore hypothyroidism is associated with increased plasma levels of cholesterol. *(Pg. 326)*

10. Which of the following is most likely to bring about improvements in exophthalmos?

A. Administration of T_4
B. Administration of drugs that inhibit the production of T lymphocytes
C. Administration of testosterone

D. Hypophysectomy
E. Thyroidectomy

Ans. (B)

Explanation:

(Pg. 39)

- **Graves' disease is an autoimmune** disease in which antibodies to TSH receptor stimulate receptor. These substances are immunoglobin antibodies that bind with the same membrane receptors that bind TSH. They induce continual activation of cAMP system of cells, leading to hyperthyroidism. These antibodies are called thyroid stimulating immunoglobins and are designated as (TSI).

(Guyton, Pg. 940)

- **Exopthalamos** is due to swelling of retroorbital tissues and degenerative changes in extraocular muscles. (A subpopulation of fibroblasts in the orbits develop into adipocytes and their preadipocyte fibroblasts contain TSH receptor protein). The current theory of the development of exophthalamos is that when stimulated by the TSH receptor stimulating antibodies in the **circulation**, these cells release cytokines that **promote** inflammation and edema. So can be treated by drugs that inhibit production of T-lymphocytes.

11. Which of the following are *incorrectly* paired?

A. Type 1 (insulin-dependent) diabetes mellitus: antibodies against B cells
B. Myasthenia gravis: antibodies against nicotinic acetylcholine receptors
C. Multiple sclerosis: antibodies against TSH
D. Hashimoto's thyroiditis: antibodies myelin
E. Graves' disease: antibodies that stimulate TSH receptors

Ans. (D)

Explanation:

Hashimoto's thyroiditis is due to antibodies against thyroglobulin (TG) and thyroid peroxide (TP).

12. Thyroid hormone receptors bind to DNA in which of the following forms?

A. A heterodimer with the prolactin receptor
B. A heterodimer with the growth hormone receptor
C. A heterodimer with the retinoid X receptor
D. A heterodimer with the insulin receptor
E. A heterodimer with the progesterone receptor

Ans. **(C)**

Explanation:

Thyroid hormones enter cells and T_3 binds to thyroid receptors (TR) in the nuclei, T_4 can also bind but not as avidly. The hormone receptor complex then binds to DNA via zinc fingers. TRs bind to DNA as monomers homodimers and heterodimers with other nuclear receptors particularly the retinoid X receptor (RXR).

(Pg. 323)

13. Increasing intracellular I^- due to the action of the Na^+/I^- symporter is an example of:

A. Endocytosis
B. Passive diffusion
C. Na^+ and K^+ cotransport
D. Primary active transport
E. Secondary active transport

Ans. **(E)**

Explanation:

The thyroid cell membranes facing the capillaries contain a symporter/iodide pump that transports Na^+ and I^- into the cells of against an electrochemical gradient for I^-. This Na^+/I^- (NIS) symporter is capable of producing I^- concentration 30-40 times as great as the concentration in plasma.

The process involved is **secondary active transport** with the energy provided by transport of Na^+ out of thyroid cells by Na^+-K^+ ATPase$^-$. I^- moves by diffusion. *(Pg. 319)*

14. Food intake in myxedema is:

A. Greater than food intake in thyrotoxicosis
B. Same as food intake in thyrotoxicosis
C. Less than food intake in thyrotoxicosis

Ans. (C)

Explanation:

Metabolic rate is increased by T_3 and T_4, so calorogenesis is increased. *(Pg. 324)*

15. Number of α-MHC molecules in the heart in myxedema is:

A. Greater than number of MHC molecules in the heart in thyrotoxicosis
B. Same as number of α-MHC molecules in the heart in thyrotoxicosis
C. Less than number of α-MHC molecules in the heart in thyrotoxicosis

Ans. (C)

Explanation:

- The heart contains two myosin heavy chain isoforms (α-MHC and β-MHC).
- α–MHC predominates in atria in adults and its level is increased by treatment with thyroid hormones. This increases the speed of cardiac contraction.
- Conversely expression of α-MHC gene is depressed and that of β–MHC is enhanced in hypothyroidism. *(Pg. 325)*

16. Amount of endocytosis at the colloid-thyroid cell border following injection of TSH is:

A. Greater than the amount of endocytosis at the colloid-thyroid cell border following injection of T_4

B. Same as the amount of endocytosis at the colloid-thyroid cell border following injection of T_4

C. Less than the amount of endocytosis at the colloid-thyroid cell border following injection of T_4

Ans. (A)

Explanation:

TSH also known as thyrotropin, its specific actions on thyroid gland are as follows:

1. Increased proteolysis of the thyroglobulin.
2. Increased activity of the iodine pump.
3. Increased iodination of tyrosine to form thyroid hormones.
4. Increased size and increased secretory activity of thyroid cells.
5. Increased number of thyroid cells

- **Mode Action:** Via cAMP activation.

Binding of TSH with TSH receptors on cell membrane of thyroid cells

↓

Activation of adenylyl cyclase in membrane

↓

Increases formation of cAMP inside cells

↓

Activation of protein kinase

↓

Phosphorylation inside cell

↓

Increased secretion of **thyroid hormones and growth of thyroid** glandular tissue.

(Guyton, Pg. 938)

Chapter 19 Endocrine Functions of the Pancreas and the Regulation of Carbohydrate Metabolism

1. Which of the following are *incorrectly* paired?

A. B cells: insulin
B. D cells: somatostatin
C. A cells: glucagon
D. Pancreatic exocrine cells: chymotrypsinogen
E. F cells: gastrin

Ans. (E)

Explanation:

Cells in the islets can be divided into types on the basis of their staining properties and morphology. Humans have at least 4 distinct cell types:

A cells secrete	: Glucagon
B cells secrete	: Insulin
D cells secrete	: Somatostatin
E cells secrete	: Pancreatic polypeptide

2. Which of the following are incorrectly paired?

A. Epinephrine: increased glycogenolysis in skeletal muscle
B. Insulin: increased gluconeogensis
C. Glucagon: increased gluconeogenesis
D. Progesterone: increased plasma glucose level
E. Growth hormone: increased plasma glucose level

Ans. (D)

Explanation:

Progesterone has no effect on glucose level.

3. Which of the following would be *least* likely to be seen 14 days after a rat is injected with a drug that kills all of its pancreatic B cells?

A. A rise in the plasma H^+ concentration
B. A rise in the plasma glucagon concentration

C. A fall in the plasma HCO_3^+ concentration
D. A fall in the plasma amino acid concentration
E. A rise in plasma osmolality

Ans. (D)

Explanation:

The supply of amino acids is increased by gluconeogenesis, because in absence of insulin, less protein synthesis occurs in muscle, hence blood amino acid levels rise. *(Pg. 342)*

4. Glucagon is not normally found in the:

A. Brain
B. Pancreas
C. Gastrointestinal tract
D. Plasma
E. Adrenal glands

Ans. (E)

Explanation:

Human glucagon is produced by A cells of the pancreatic islets and the upper GIT. It is also found in brain. *(Pg. 348)*

5. When the plasma glucose concentration falls to low levels, a number of different hormones help combat the hypoglycemia. After intravenous administration of a large dose of insulin, the return of a low blood sugar level to normal delayed in:

A. Adrenal medullary insufficiency
B. Glucagon deficiency
C. Combined adrenal medullary insufficiency and glucagon deficiency
D. Thyrotoxicosis
E. Acromegaly

Ans. (C)

Explanation:

Many hormones in addition to insulin, IGF-I and

IGF-II have important roles in the regulation of carbohydrate metabolism. They include glucagon, epinephrine, thyroid hormones, glucocorticoids and growth hormones. *(Pg. 351)*

6. Which of the following is not produced by total pancreatectomy?

A. Steatorrhea
B. Increased plasma levels of free fatty acids
C. Decreased plasma PCO_2
D. No change or a rise in the plasma insulin level
E. No change or a rise in the plasma glucagon level

Ans. (D)

Explanation:

Removal of pancreas will lead to removal of B cells, which are the source of insulin.

7. Insulin increases the entry of glucose into:

A. All tissues
B. Renal tubular cells
C. The mucosa in the small intestine
D. Most neurons in the cerebral cortex
E. Skeletal muscle

Ans. (E)

Explanation:

In Muscle – Fat – Some other tissues	**Insulin facilitates glucose** entry into cells by increasing number of glucose transporters in the cell membranes while in
– Intestine and Kidneys	Glucose enters cells by secondary active transport with Na^+

(Pg. 336)

8. The mechanism by which glucagon produces an increase in the plasma glucose concentration involves:

A. Binding of glucagon to DNA in the nucleus of target cells
B. Binding of glucagon to receptors in the cytoplasm of target cells
C. Activation of G_s in target cells
D. Increased binding of Ca^{2+} in the cytoplasm of target cells
E. Inhibition of insulin secretion

Ans. (C) *(Pg. 348)*

Explanation:

- Glucagon acts on serpentine receptors. It acts via G_S to activate **adenylyl cyclase** and increases **protein kinase A** which increases phosphorylation leading to increase in **glycogenolysis** which increases blood glucose levels.
(Fig. 19.16, Pg. 349)
- Glucagon does not cause glycogenolysis in muscle. It increases glycogenolysis only in liver.

9. Glucagon increases glycogenolysis in liver cells but ACTH does not because:

A. Cortisol increases the plasma glucose level
B. Liver cells have an adenylyl cyclase different from that in adrenocortical cells
C. ACTH cannot enter the nucleus of liver cells
D. The membranes of liver cells contain receptors different from those in adrenocortical cells
E. Liver cells contain a protein that inhibits the action of ACTH

Ans. (D)

Explanation:

- The membranes of liver cells contain receptors different from those in adrenocortical cells.

- Glucocorticoids are necessary for the glucagon to exert its gluconeogenic action during fasting. They are gluconeogenic themselves, but their role is mainly permissive. The major diabetogenic effects are an:
  1. Increase in protein catabolism with increased gluconeogenesis in liver and ketogenesis.
  2. Decrease in peripheral glucose utilization relative to the blood insulin level that may be due to inhibition of glucose phosphorylation.

10. A meal rich in proteins containing the amino acids that stimulate insulin secretion but low in carbohydrate does not cause hypoglycemia because:

A. The meal causes a compensatory increase in T_4 secretion
B. Cortisol in the circulation prevents glucose from entering muscle
C. Glucagon secretion is also stimulated by the meal
D. The amino acids in the meal are promptly converted to glucose
E. Insulin does not bind to insulin receptors if the plasma concentration of amino acids is elevated

Ans. (C)

Explanation:

Insulin is	- Glycogenic
Hormone of energy	- Antigluconeogenitic
storage	- Antilipolytic
	- Antiketotic
Glucagon on the other hand is:	- Glycogenolytic
Hormone of energy release.	- Gluconeogenic
	- Lipolytic
	- Ketogenic

- Insulin-glucagon molar ratios fluctuate markedly because the secretion of glucagon and insulin are both modified by various conditions e.g. insulin-glucagon molar ratio an a balanced diet is $\simeq$ 2.3.

11. Glucose increases plasma insulin by a process that involves:

- **A.** GLUT 1
- **B.** GLUT 2
- **C.** GLUT 3
- **D.** GLUT 4
- **E.** SGLT 1

Ans. (B)

Explanation:

GLUT-2 is B-cell glucose sensor.

12. Insulin secretion after glucose is given intravenously is:

- **A.** Greater than insulin secretion after the same amount of glucose is given orally
- **B.** Same as insulin secretion after the same amount of glucose is given orally
- **C.** Less than insulin secretion after the same amount of glucose is given orally

Ans. (C)

Explanation:

- Orally administered glucose exerts a greater insulin stimulating effect than intravenously administered glucose and orally administered amino acids also produce a greater insulin response than intravenous amino acids. These observations led to exploration of the possibility that a substance secreted by the gastrointestinal mucosa stimulated insulin secretion.
- Glucagon, glucagon-derivatives, secretin, cholecystokinin (CCK), gastrin and gastric inhibitory peptide (GIP), all have such an action and CCK potentiates the insulin stimulating effects of amino acids.
- Recently glucagon-like peptide (GLP-1) is considered an additional gut factor that stimulates insulin secretion.

13. Plasma glucose level after surgical pancreatectomy is:

A. Greater than plasma glucose level after administration of a toxin such as alloxan that selectively kills B cells

B. Same as plasma glucose level after administration of a toxin such as alloxan that selectively kills B cells

C. Less than plasma glucose level after administration of a toxin such as alloxan that selectively kills B cells

Ans. (C)

Explanation:

Glucagon is spared by alloxan, while pancreatomy removes whole of pancreas.

14. Plasma concentration of C peptide in fasting subject is:

A. Greater than plasma concentration of C peptide in fed state

B. Same as plasma concentration of C peptide in fed state

C. Less than plasma concentration of C peptide in fed state

Ans. (C)

Explanation:

The peptide segment connecting A and B chains (connecting peptide, C peptide) facilitates the folding and then is detached in the granules before secretion. Normally 90-97% of the product is released from B cells is insulin also along with the equimolar amounts of C peptide can be measured by radioimmunoassay and its level provides an index of B cell function in patients receiving exogenous insulin.

UNIT IV. ENDOCRINOLOGY, METABOLISM AND REPRODUCTIVE FUNCTION

Chapter 20 The Adrenal Medulla and Adrenal Cortex

1. Which of the following is produced only by *large amounts* of glucocorticoids?

A. Normal responsiveness of fat depots to norepinephrine
B. Maintenance of normal vascular reactivity
C. Increased excretion of a water load
D. Inhibition of the inflammatory response
E. Inhibition of ACTH secretion

Ans. (D)

Explanation:

Glucocorticoids inhibit the inflammatory response to tissue injury. They also suppress manifestations of allergic disease that are due to release of histamine from tissues. Both of these effects require high levels of circulating glucocorticoids and cannot be produced by administering steroids without producing the other manifestations of glucocorticoid excess. *(Pg. 371)*

2. Which of the following are *incorrectly* paired?

A. Gluconeogenesis: cortisol
B. Free fatty acid mobilization: dehydroepiandrosterone
C. Muscle glycogenolysis: epinephrine
D. Kaliuresis: aldosterone
E. Hepatic glycogenesis: insulin

Ans. (B)

Explanation:

Androgens are the hormones that exert masculinizing effects and they promote protein anabolism and growth. The main adrenal androgens are **dehydroepiandrosterone (DHEA)** and **androstenedione.** *(Pg. 368)*

3. **Which of the following hormones has the shortest plasma half-life?**
   A. Corticosterone
   B. Renin
   C. Dehydroepiandrosterone
   D. Aldosterone
   E. Norepinephrine

Ans. (E)

Explanation:

Plasma ½ life of corticosterone	:	50 min (Pg 366)
Plasma ½ life of renin in circulation	:	80 min or less (Pg 454)
Plasma ½ life of aldosterone	:	20 min (Pg 367)
Plasma ½ life of NE (For all catecholamines)	:	2 min (Pg 358)
Plasma ½ life of Dehydroepiandrosterone	:	12 hours

4. **Mole for mole, which of the following has the greatest effect on Na^+ excretion?**
   A. Progesterone
   B. Cortisol
   C. Vasopressin
   D. Aldosterone
   E. Dehydroepiandrosterone

Ans. (D)

Explanation:

Aldosterone and other steroids with mineralocorticoid activity increases reabsorption of Na^+ from urine, saliva, sweat and the contents of urine. Thus mineralocorticoids cause retention of Na^+ in ECF. *(Pg. 375, 380)*

5. Mole for mole, which of the following has the greatest effect on plasma osmolality?

A. Progesterone
B. Cortisol
C. Vasopressin
D. Aldosterone
E. Dehydroepiandrosterone

Ans. (C)

Explanation:

Vasopressin secretion is controlled by a delicate feedback mechanism that operates continuously to defend the osmolality of the plasma, which is maintained very close to 285 mosm/l. *(Pg. 245)*

6. The secretion of which of the following would be *least* affected by a decrease in extracellular fluid volume?

A. CRH
B. Arginine vasopressin
C. Dehydroepiandrosterone
D. Estrogens
E. Aldosterone

Ans. (D)

7. A young man presents with a blood pressure of 175/110 mmHg. He is found to have a high circulating aldosterone but a low circulating cortisol.
Glucocorticoid treatment lowers his circulating aldosterone and lowers his blood pressure to 140/85 mmHg. He probably has an abnormal:

A. 17 α-hydroxylase
B. 21 β-hydroxylase
C. 3 β-hydroxysteroid dehydrogenase
D. Aldosterone synthase
E. Cholesterone desmolase

Ans. (D)

(Guyton, Pg. 946)

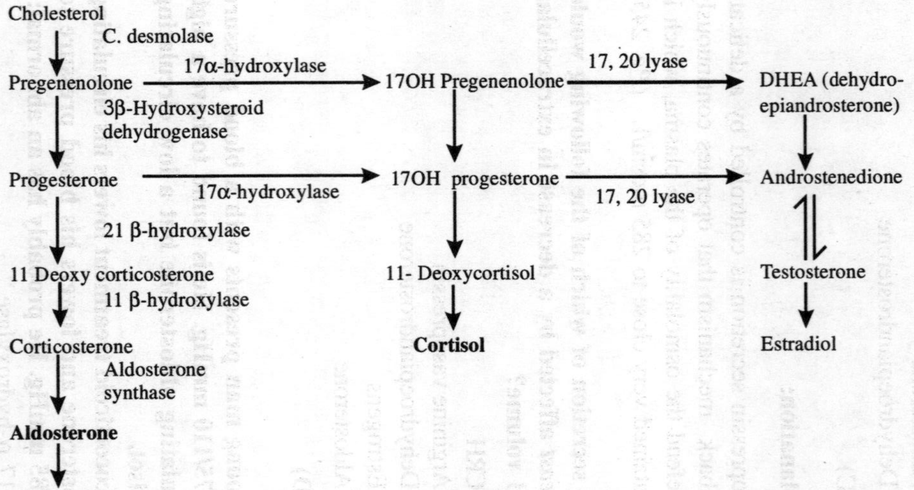

Guyton, Pg 946 (11th edition).
Hormone synthesis in zona fasciculata and zona reticularis of adrenal cortex.
In **zona glomerulosa**, there is no **11 β-hydroxylase, instead there is aldosterone synthase.** (Pg. 364)

Cholesterol
↓ ACTH, AII
Pregnenolone
↓
Progesterone
(Pregnenolone, Progesterone → Cortisol and sex steroids.)
↓
Deoxycorticosterone
↓ Aldosterone synthase
Corticosterone
↓ Aldosterone synthase, AII
18-hydroxycorticosterone
↓ Aldosterone synthase
Aldosterone

Hormone synthesis in zona glomerulosa

Aldosterone synthase is found only in zona glomerulosa. This zona also lacks 17α-hydroxylase. This is why the zona glomerulosa makes aldosterone but fails to make cortisol/sex hormones.

8. A 32-year-old woman presents with a blood pressure of 155/96 mmHg. In response to questioning, she admits that she loves licorice and eats some at least three times a week. She probably has a low level of:

A. Type 2 11 β-hydroxysteroid dehydrogenase activity
B. ACTH
C. 11 β-hydroxylase activity
D. Glucuronyl transferase
E. Norepinephrine

Ans. (A)

Explanation:

***See* Flow Chart 2 on the next page**

Metabolism and excretion of glucocorticoids hepatic metabolism

Cortisol → Dihydrocortisol → **Tetrahydrocortisol** → **Tetrahydrocortisol glucuronide**

Cortisol → **17-ketosteroids**

11β-hydroxysteroid dehydrogenase: **Cortisol** ⇄ **Cortisone**

Cortisone → **17-ketosteroids**

- Liver and other tissues contain the enzyme **11β-hydroxysteroid dehydrogenase.** There are two forms of this enzyme.

Form 1:
Catalyzes conversion of
cortisol ⇄ cortisone and reverse

Form 2:
Exclusive conversion of
cortisol → cortisone

(Pg. 368, 376)

Mineralocorticoid receptors have high affinity for glucocorticoids and glucocorticoid receptors has. So why glucocorticoids donot bind to mineralocorticoid receptors in kidneys and other locations and produce mineralocorticoid effects. The reason is that kidneys and other mineralocorticoid sensitive tissues also contain enzyme **11 β-hydroxysteroid dehydrogenase type 2.** This leaves aldosterone untouched, but converts cortisol to cortisone.

i.e. Cortisol

↓

Cortisone

↓

11 Oxyderivative → donot bind to receptors

- If 11 β hydroxysteroid dehydrogenase type 2 is inhibited or absent, cortisol has marked mineralocorticoid effects. The resulting syndrome is called apparent **mineralocorticoid excess (AME).**
- This can be congenital or prolonged ingestion of licorice, which contains glycyrrhetinic acid which inhibits the enzyme.

9. Which of the following is *not* characteristic of primary hyperaldosteroidism?

A. Low plasma renin activity
B. Normal plasma ACTH
C. Hypertension
D. High plasma Na^+
E. Low plasma K^+

Ans. (D)

Explanation:

Primary Hyperaldosteronism/Conn's Syndrome *(Pg. 380)*

Seen in:

- Adenoma of zona glomerulosa.
- Unilateral/bilateral adrenal hyperplasia.

- Tumor is secreting large amounts of aldosterone.

Clinical Features

- Renin secretion is depressed (diagnostic criteria).
- Na^+ retention, K^+ depletion (hypokalemia, weakness).
- Hypertension.
- No edema.

Secondary Hyperaldosteronism is having:

- High renin activity.

Seen in:

- Cirrhosis.
- Heart failure.
- Nephrosis (leading to high renin).

10. In its action on cells, aldosterone:

A. Increases transport of ENaCs from the cytoplasm to the cell membrane
B. Does not act on the cell membrane
C. Binds to a receptor in the nucleus
D. May activate a heat shock protein
E. Also binds to glucocorticoid receptors

Ans. (A)

Like many steroids, aldosterone binds to cytoplamic receptor→receptor hormone complex→binds to nucleus→alters transcription of mRNA's →increases production of proteins→proteins alter cell function.

Aldosterone stimulated proteins have 2 actions:

Fast action	**Slow action**
Increasing activity of epithelial sodium channels (ENaCs) by Insertion of these channels form cytoplasmic pool into cell membrane	Increases synthesis of ENaCs

(Pg. 375)

UNIT IV. ENDOCRINOLOGY, METABOLISM AND REPRODUCTIVE FUNCTION

Chapter 21 Hormonal Control of Calcium Metabolism and the Physiology of Bone

1. A patient with parathyroid deficiency 10 days after inadvertent damage to the parathyroid glands during thyroid surgery would probably have:

A. Low plasma phosphate and Ca^{2+} levels and tetany

B. Low plasma phosphate and Ca^{2+} levels and tetanus

C. A low plasma Ca^{2+} level, increased muscular excitability, and a characteristic spasm of the muscles of the upper extremity (Trousseau's sign)

D. High plasma phosphate Ca^{2+} levels and bone demineralization

E. Increased muscular excitability, a high plasma Ca^{2+} level, and bone demineralization

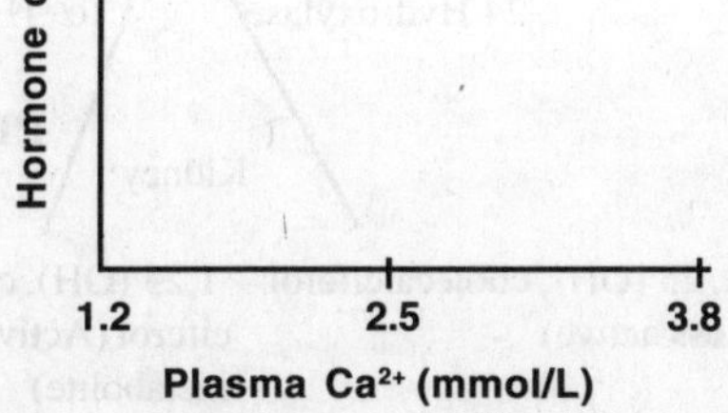

Ans. (C)

Explanation:

In humans, tetany is most often due to inadvertent parathyroidectomy during thyroid surgery.

Symptoms usually develop 2-3 days post-operatively but may not appear for several weeks or more. The signs of tetany in humans include **Trousseau's sign,** a spasm of muscles of upper extremity that causes flexion of wrist and thumb with extension of fingers. *(Pg. 392)*

2. A high plasma Ca^{2+} level causes:

A. Bone demineralization
B. Increased formation of 1, 25-dihydroxy-cholecalciferol
C. Decreased secretion of calcitonin
D. Decreased blood coagulability
E. Increased formation of 24, 25-dihydroxy-cholecalciferol

Ans. (E)

Explanation:

<u>Formation and hydroxylation of Vit D_3</u>

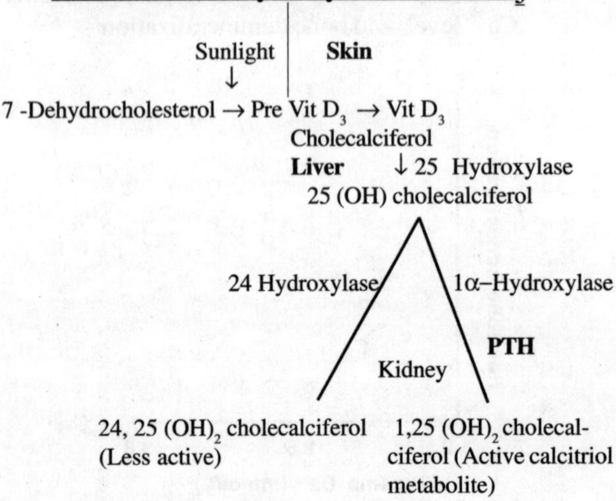

- Production of 1,25 $(OH)_2$ cholecalciferol is increased by low Ca^{+2} and inhibited by high plasma PO_4^{3-} levels.
- Additional control of its production is exerted by a direct:
  1. Negative feedback of the metabolite on 1α hydroxylase.
  2. The feedback action on formation of 24, 25 $(OH)_2$ cholecalciferol.
  3. Direct action on parathyroid gland to inhibit the production of mRNA for PTH.

Feedback control of formation of 1,25(OH)D_3 in kidneys.

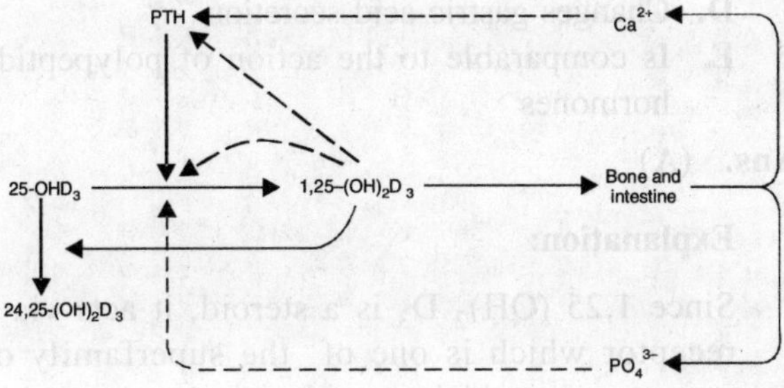

(Pg. 389)

3. Which of the following is *not* involved in regulating plasma Ca^{2+} levels?

A. Kidneys
B. Skin
C. Liver
D. Lungs
E. Intestine

Ans. (D) Lungs (See Ans. 2)

4. Which of the following exerts the greatest effect on parathyroid hormone secretion?

A. Plasma phosphate concentration
B. Calcitonin
C. 1, 25-Dihydroxycholecalciferol
D. Total plasma calcium concentration
E. Plasma Ca^{2+} concentration

Ans. (E)

Explanation:

See Flow Chart of Ans. No.2 (Feedback control) Circulating ionized Ca^{+2} acts directly on the parathyroid gland in a negative feedback to regulate secretion of PTH.

- Key to this regulation is a cell membrane Ca^{+2} receptor. *(Pg. 392)*

5. 1, 25-Dihydroxycholecalciferol affects intestinal Ca^{2+} absorption through a mechanism that:

A. Includes alterations in the activity of genes
B. Activates adenylyl cyclase
C. Decreases cell turnover
D. Changes gastric acid secretion
E. Is comparable to the action of polypeptide hormones

Ans. (A)

Explanation:

Since 1,25 $(OH)_2$ D_3 is a steroid, it acts via a receptor which is one of the superfamily of receptors, by which steroids, trigger changes in gene expression.

- Binding of steroid to receptors–exposes DNA binding region–increased transcription of some mRNA. Calbindin D proteins in case of 1,25 $(OH)_2$ D_3 and inhibition of transcription of others.
- Calbindin D proteins are members of superfamily of Ca^{+2} binding proteins. Found in intestine, brain and kidneys. *(Pg. 388)*

6. Which of the following would you expect to find in a patient whose diet has been low in calcium for 2 months?

A. Increased formation of 24, 25-dihydroxychole-calciferol
B. Decreased amounts of calcium-binding protein in intestinal epithelial cells
C. Increased parathyroid hormone secretion

D. A high plasma calcitonin concentration
E. Increased plasma phosphates

Ans. (C)

Explanation:

See Ans. 2 and Ans. 4

Plasma Ca^{+2} **ion has greatest effect on parathyroid hormone secretion.**

7. A 57-year-old woman complains of fatigue and weight loss. She has an elevated plasma Ca^{2+}, but her plasma PTH is zero. The most likely diagnosis is:

A. A gain-of-function mutation of the gene coding Ca^{2+} receptors
B. Adrenal insufficiency
C. Hypoparathyroidism
D. Hypopituitarism
E. Cancer of the colon

Ans. (E)

Explanation:

Hypercalcaemia is a common metabolic complication of cancer. About 20% of hypercalcaemia patients have bone metastases that produce hypercalcaemia by eroding bone (*local osteolytic hypercalcaemia*). Erosion is produced by PGE (Prostaglandins) from tumor.

- Tumors responsible for hypersecretion include cancers of breast, kidney, ovary and skin.

(Pg. 393)

8. In which of the following diseases is plasma PTH often elevated?

A. Pseudohypoparathyroidism
B. Adrenal failure
C. Cancer
D. Congestive heart failure
E. Precocious puberty

Ans. (A)

Explanation:

In disease of **pseudohypoparathyroidism**, signs and symptoms of hypoparathyoidism develop but the circulating level of PTH is normal or elevated. Since, the tissues fail to respond, to this hormone, this is a receptor disease. *(Pg. 391)*

9. In osteogenesis imperfecta, which of the following is defective?

A. Phosphate deposition in trabecular bone
B. Structure of PTHrP
C. Osteoblasts
D. Osteoclasts
E. Bone collagen

Ans. (E)

Explanation:

In osteogenesis imperfecta (brittle bone disease) various mutations in the genes that code for collagen make bones brittle, so collagen is defective. *(Pg. 386)*

10. In osteopetrosis, which of the following is defective?

A. Phosphate deposition in trabecular bone
B. Structure of PTHrP
C. Osteoblasts
D. Osteoclasts
E. Bone collagen

Ans. (D)

Explanation:

Osteopetrosis: Osteoclasts are defective and are unable to resorb bone in their usual fashion so osteoblasts operate unopposed. The result is:

1. Steady increase in **bone density.**
2. **Neurologic defects** due to narrowing and distortion of foramina through which nerves normally pass; and

3. **Haematologic abnormalities** due to crowding out of marrow cavities. *(Pg. 386)*

11. PTH and PTHrP activate the same receptor, but their effects are different. Which of the following is the most likely explanation of this observation?

A. For unknown reasons, PTHrP acts mainly on fetal tissues, whereas PTH acts mainly on adult tissues

B. Plasma PTH is high when plasma PTHrP is low and vice versa

C. PTH acts on the brain, whereas PTHrP does not

D. When PTH binds to the common receptor, it activates adenylyl cyclase, whereas PTHrP activates phospholipase C

E. There is an additional receptor in the body that responds to PTH but not to PTHrP

Ans. (E)

Explanation:

A protein with PTH activity, i.e., parathyroid hormone related protein (PTHrP) is produced by many different tissues in body.

- Both PTH and PTHrP bind to same receptor, both effects are different because:
  - PTHrP is primarily a tissue hormone or factor, acting where it is produced, it may be that circulating PTH cannot reach these sites.
  - Another possibility is action of one or the other hormone on other, more selective receptors.

(Pg. 393)

12. Percentage of increased Ca^{2+} absorbed from the intestine in a subject fed is:

A. Greater than the percentage of ingested Ca^{2+} absorbed from the intestine in a subject fed a low-calcium diet

B. Same as the percentage of ingested Ca^{2+} absorbed from the intestine in a subject fed a low-calcium diet

C. Less than the percentage of ingested Ca^{2+} absorbed from the intestine in a subject fed a low-calcium diet

Ans. (C)

Explanation:

When Ca^{2+} intake is high, – 1,25 $(OH)_2$ D_3 levels fall because of increased plasma Ca^{2+}. Consequently Ca^{2+} absorption undergoes adaptation, i.e., high when Ca intake is low and decrease when Ca intake is high. *(Pg. 382)*

13. Concentration of PTHrP in milk is:

A. Greater than the concentration of PTHrP in plasma collected at the same time

B. Same as the concentration of PTHrP in plasma collected at the same time

C. Less than the concentration of PTHrP in plasma collected at the same time

Ans. (A)

Explanation:

In normal lactating mice, there is abundant PTHrP in milk. However, plasma level does not increase during lactation and the function of PTHrP in milk is unknown. *(Pg. 393)*

Chapter 22 Pituitary Gland

1. Which of the following hormones exerts the least effect on growth?

A. Growth hormones
B. Testosterone
C. T_4
D. Insulin
E. Vasopressin

Ans. (E)

Explanation:

Vasopressin is mainly responsible for maintenance of plasma osmolality at 285 mosm/l, so its principal physiologic effect is retention of water by the kidney. *(Pg. 244-245)*

2. Which of the following are *incorrectly* paired?

A. Intermediate lobe: corticotrophin-like intermediate lobe peptide (CLIP)
B. Hypothyroidism: low plasma growth hormone concentration
C. Gigantism: increased growth hormone secretion before puberty
D. African pygmies: low plasma growth hormone
E. Acromegaly: high plasma IGF-I concentration

Ans. (D)

Explanation:

African pygmies have normal plasma growth hormone levels, and a modest reduction in the plasma of GH binding protein. Their plasma IGF-I (insulin growth factor-I) fails to increase at the time of puberty. *(Pg. 407)*

3. Which of the following pituitary hormones is an opioid peptide?

A. α-Melanocyte-stimulating hormone (α-MSH)
B. β-MSH
C. ACTH
D. Growth hormone
E. β-endorphin

Ans. (E)

Explanation:

Intermediate lobe cells and **corticotropes** of the anterior lobe both synthesize a large percursor protein. This prohormone is known as proopiomelanocortin (POMC). This molecule is also synthesized in the hypothalamus, the lungs, the gastrointestinal tract and the placenta. In the corticotropes, it is hydrolyzed to ACTH and βLPH plus a small amount of β-endorphin and these substances are secreted.

In **intermediate lobe cells**: POMC is further hydrolyzed to corticotropin like intermediate lobe peptide (CLIP), γ-LPH and appreciable amounts of β-endorphin (opoid peptide). The functions of CLIP and γ-LPH are unknown, while β-endorphin is an opoid peptide.

4. Which of the following hormones is *not* made up of α and β subunits?

A. TSH
B. LH
C. FSH
D. hCG
E. Prolactin

Ans. (E)

Explanation:

FSH and LH, TSH and HCG are each made up of an α and β subunits. ACTH, prolactin and growth hormone (GH) are simple polypeptides or proteins. Human prolaction has considerable structural similarity to human GH and hCS.

(Pg. 396,421,422)

5. **Which of the following in *not* characteristic of hypopituitarism?**
   A. Cachexia
   B. Infertility
   C. Pallor
   D. Low basal metabolic rate
   E. Intolerance to stress

Ans. (A)

Explanation:

Loss of GH causes loss of body protein and increased body fat along with decreased vitality. There may be some loss of protein in adults but wasting is not a feature of hypopituitarism in humans and most patients with pituitary insufficiency are well nourished. *(Pg. 409)*

6. **Which of the following in *not* synthesized in both endocrine glands and the brain?**
   A. Somatostatin
   B. Cortisol
   C. Dopamine
   D. ACTH
   E. ERβ

Ans. (B)

Explanation:

Cortisol is formed by adrenal cortex.
Estrogen receptor β is found primarily in the ovaries, prostrate, lungs, GIT tract and CNS. *(Pg. 442)*

Somatostatin is found in various parts of the brain where it functions as a neurotransmitter. In the hypothalamus it is growth hormone inhibiting hormone secreted into the portal hypophysial vessels, in the endocrine pancreas it inhibits insulin secretion and the secretion of various pancreatic hormones and in GIT it is important inhibitory gastrointestinal hormone.

ACTH is secreted by anterior pituitary.
Dopamine: There are many dopaminergic systems in the brain and is also secreted by adrenal medulla.

7. A scientist finds that infusion of growth hormone into the median eminence of the hypothalamus in experimental animals inhibits the secretion of growth hormone, and concludes that this proves that growth hormone feeds back to inhibit GRH secretion. Do you accept this conclusion?

A. No, because growth hormone does not cross the blood-brain barrier
B. No, because the infused growth hormone could be stimulating dopamine secretion
C. No, because substances placed in the median eminence could be transported to the anterior pituitary
D. Yes, because systemically administered growth hormone inhibits growth hormone secretion
E. Yes, because growth hormone binds GRH, inactivating it

Ans. (C)

8. The growth hormone receptor:

A. Activates G_s
B. Requires dimerization to exert its effects
C. Must be internalized to exert its effects
D. Resembles the IGF-I receptor
E. Resembles the ACTH receptor

Ans. (B)

Explanation:

Growth hormone receptor has a:

1. Large extracellular portion.
2. A transmembrane domain.
3. A large cytoplasmic portion.
   - It is a member of cytokine receptor superfamily.

- GH has 2 binding sites for receptors, when it binds to one of the receptor subunits, the other binding site attracts another subunit, producing a homodimer. **Dimerization is essential for receptor activation.** *(Pg. 400)*

9. Achondroplasia is due to:

A. Fibroblast growth factor receptor 3 gene defect
B. Chronic abuse and neglect
C. Defective growth hormone receptors
D. Thyroid hormone deficiency
E. Increased circulating gonadal steroids

Ans. (A)

Explanation:

- Achondroplasia is most common form of dwarfism in humans and is characterized by short limbs with a normal trunk.
- It is **autosomonal dominant** condition caused by mutation in the gene that codes for **fibroblast growth factor receptor 3 (FGFR3)**. This receptor is normally expressed in cartilage and bone. *(Pg. 408)*

10. Plasma growth hormone (GH) level after 30 minutes of sleep is:

A. Greater than plasma growth hormone level after 8 hours of sleep
B. Same as plasma growth hormone level after 8 hours of sleep
C. Less than plasma growth hormone level after 8 hours of sleep

Ans. (A)

Explanation:

A spike in GH secretion occurs with considerable regularity on going to sleep. *(Pg. 403)*

11. Insulin sensitivity in hypopituitarism is:

A. Greater than insulin sensitivity in acromegaly

B. Same as insulin sensitivity in acromegaly

C. Less than insulin sensitivity in acromegaly

Ans. (A)

Explanation:

Hypopituitarism increases sensitivity to insulin because they lack the anti-insulin effects of growth hormone (GH). *(Pg. 400)*

Chapter 23 The Gonads: Development and Function of the Reproductive System

In questions 1-5 refer to figure below:

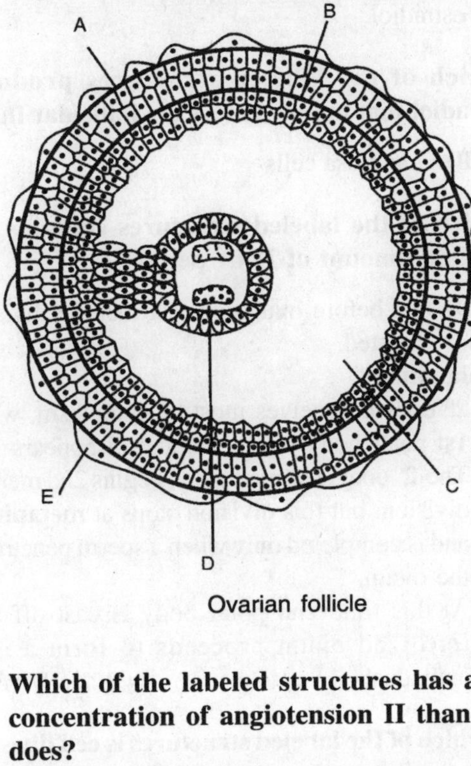

Ovarian follicle

1. Which of the labeled structures has a higher concentration of angiotension II than plasma does?

Ans. (C)

Explanation:

There are AT_2 receptors, which are coded in humans by a gene on the X chromosome. AT_2 receptors are more plentiful in fetal and neonatal life, but they persist in the brain and other organs in adults. *(Pg. 457)*

2. Which of the labeled structures produces the most androstenedione?

Ans. (A) *(Fig. 23.30, Pg. 440)*

Explanation:

- Theca interna cells have many LH receptors and LH acts via cAMP to increase conversion of cholesterol to androstenedione.
- Theca interna cells also supply androstenedione to granulosa cells, then granulosa cells make estradiol.

3. Which of the labeled structures produces estradiol that mainly enters the follicular fluid?

Ans. **(B)** Granulosa cells

4. Which of the labeled structures contains the smallest amount of DNA per cell?

Ans. **(D)** Just before ovulation, 1st meiotic division is completed.

Explanation:

- 2° oocyte, receives most of cytoplasm, while 1st polar body fragments and disappears.
- The 2° oocyte immediately, begins 2nd meiotic division, but this division stops at **metaphase** and is completed only when a sperm penetrates the ovum.
- At this time 2nd polar body is cast off and fertilized ovum proceeds to form a new individual. *(Pg. 435)*

5. In which of the labeled structures is cell division arrested in prophase?

Ans. **(D)** It has not got ovulated. After ovulation, 2° oocyte is formed.

Explanation:

At the time of birth, there are 2 million ova, but 50% of these are atretic. The million that are normal undergo the first part of the 1st meiotic division at about this time and enter a stage of arrest in prophase in which those that survive persist until adulthood.

(See also Ans. 4)

6. If a young woman has high plasma levels of T_3, cortisol, and renin activity but her blood pressure is only slightly elevated and she has no symptoms or signs of thyrotoxicosis or Cushing's syndrome, the most likely explanation is that:

A. She has been treated with TSH and ACTH
B. She has been treated with T_3 and cortisol
C. She is in the third trimester of pregnancy
D. She has an adrenocortical tumor
E. She has been subjected to chronic stress

Ans. (C)

Explanation:

During pregnancy, TBG increases, also there is increase in transcortin (binding protein for cortical), so plasma T_3 and cortical increase (bound form). *(Pg. 322)*

7. Full development and function of the seminiferous tubules require:

A. Somatostatin
B. LH
C. Oxytocin
D. FSH
E. Androgens and FSH

Ans. (E)

Explanation:

The differentiation of the primitive gonads into testes or ovaries in utero is genetically determined in humans, but formation of male genitalia depends on the presence of a functional, secreting testis. When the embryo has functional testis, male external and internal genitalia develop. The leydig cells of fetal testis secrete testosterone and sertoli cells secrete MIS (Mullerian inhibiting substance). After birth, gonads remain quiescent until adolescence, when they are activated by gonadotropins from anterior pituitary. *(Pg. 411, 414)*

8. In humans, fertilization usually occurs in the:

- **A.** Vagina
- **B.** Cervix
- **C.** Uterine cavity
- **D.** Uterine tubes
- **E.** Abdominal cavity

Ans. (D)

Explanation:

In humans, fertilization of the ovum by the sperm usually occurs in the **ampulla** of the **uterine** tube. *(Pg. 448)*

9. In human males, testosterone is produced mainly by the:

- **A.** Leydig cells
- **B.** Sertoli cells
- **C.** Seminiferous tubules
- **D.** Epididymis
- **E.** Vas deferens

Ans. (A)

Explanation:

Interstitial cells of leydig secretes testosterone into the blood stream. *(Pg. 424)*

10. Home-use kits for determining a woman's fertile period depend on the detection of one hormone in the urine. This hormone is:

- **A.** FSH
- **B.** Progesterone
- **C.** Estradiol
- **D.** hCG
- **E.** LH

Ans. (E)

Explanation:

A surge in LH secretion triggers ovulation and ovulation normally occurs about **9 hours after the peak of LH surge at midcycle.**

11. Puberty does not normally occur in humans under the age of 8 years, because before that age:

A. The tissues are unresponsive to gonadal steroids
B. The ovaries and testes are unresponsive to gonadal nadotropins
C. The pituitary cannot manufacture adequate amounts of gonadotropins
D. The brain secretes a substance that inhibits the responsiveness of the gonads to gonadotropins
E. The hypothalamus fails to secrete GnRH in a pulsatile fashion

Ans. (E)

Explanation:

During the period from birth to puberty, a neural mechanism is operating to prevent the normal pulsatile release of GnRH. The nature of mechanism inhibiting the GnRH pulse generator is unknown. However one or more genes produce products that stimulates secretion of GnRH. Thus it seems clear that pulsatile secretion of GnRH brings on puberty.

(Pg. 419)

12. Castration cells are found in the:

A. Uterus
B. Prostate
C. Placenta
D. Anterior pituitary
E. Hypothalamus

Ans. (D)

Explanation:

This term pertains to a **cell type** found in the pituitary after surgical or drug-induced castration. Castration cells may have the morphology of **signet ring cells** or appear as giant hypertrophic **cells**. They are discriminated easily from other pituitary **cells** without immunostaining.

Castration cells have been confirmed to be hyperfunctioning **gonadotropes**, which transform into castration cells, for example, after gonadectomy, or treatment with anti-androgens, gonadotropin releasing **hormone** agonists or aminoglutethimide, i.e., in strongly hyperactive states.

13. Decidual cells are found in the:

A. Uterus
B. Prostate
C. Placenta
D. Anterior pituitary
E. Hypothalamus

Ans. (A)

Explanation:

Before the fertilized **ovum** reaches the **uterus**, the **mucous membrane** of the body of the uterus undergoes important changes and is then known as the **decidua**. The thickness and vascularity of the mucous membrane are greatly increased; its glands are elongated and open on its free surface by funnel-shaped **orifices**, while their deeper portions are tortuous and dilated into irregular spaces. The interglandular tissue is also increased in quantity, and is crowded with large round, oval, or polygonal cells, termed **decidual cells**. Their enlargement is due to glycogen and lipid accumulation in the cytoplasm allowing these cells to provide a rich source of nutrition for the developing embryo.

14. Which of the following is *not* a steroid?

A. 17 α-Hydroxyprogesterone
B. Estrone
C. Relaxin
D. Pregnenolone
E. Etiocholanolone

Ans. (C)

Explanation:

Relaxin is a polypeptide, while rest are all steroids.

15. Which of the following is *not* a male secondary sexual characteristic?

A. A beard
B. An increased incidence of acne
C. A deep voice
D. Increased fat in the buttocks
E. An enlarged penis

Ans. (D)

Explanation:

Changes at puberty in boys (male secondary sexual characteristics)

1. **External genitalia**
   Penis increases in length and width.
   Scrotum becomes pigmented and rugose.
2. **Internal genitalia**
   Seminal vesicles enlarge and secrete and begin to form fructose.
   Prostate and bulbourethral glands enlarge and secrete.
3. **Voice**
   Larynx enlarges.
   Vocal cords increase in length and thickness.
   Voice deepens.
4. **Hair growth**
   Beard appears. Hairline on scalp reeds anterolaterally.
   Hair appears in axillas, on chest and around anus, general body hair increases.
5. **Mental**
   More aggressive.
   Interest in opposite sex develops.
6. **Body conformation**
   Shoulders broaden, muscles enlarge.
7. **Skin**
   Sebaceous glands secretion thickens and increases. *(Pg. 430)*

16. Sildenafil (Viagra) causes transient difficulty with color perception because:

A. It dilates the blood vessels in the retina
B. It constricts the blood vessels in the retina
C. Related isoforms of guanylyl cyclase are found in the retina and in the penis
D. Related isoforms of phosphodiesterase are found in the retina and in the penis
E. The retina and the penis arise from the same embryonic structure

Ans. (D)

Explanation:

Erection is mediated by efferent parasympathetic fibers that are present in pelvic splanchnic nerves (Nervi erigentes) and contain acetylcholine and VIP. There are also nonadrenergic noncholinergic fibers in the nervi erigentes and these contain large amounts of **NO synthase,** the enzyme that catalyzes formation of NO.

NO activates cyclase

↓

Guanylyl cyclase → GTP → cGMP leads to smooth muscle relaxation.

So NO plays an important role in the erection.

Sildenafil (Viagra) inhibits breakdown of cGMP by phosphodiesterases, so is used in treatment of impotence.

- A type of phosphodiesterase is found in retina and **Sildenafil** also produces significant inhibition of this phosphodiesterase. So one of side effects of this drug is transient loss of ability to discriminate between blue and green. *(Pg. 428)*

17. Which of the following probably triggers the onset of labor?

A. ACTH in the fetus

B. ACTH in the mother
C. Prostaglandins
D. Oxytocin
E. Placental renin

Ans. (A)

Explanation:

In humans CRH secretion by the fetal hypothalamus increases, and is supplemented by increased placental production of CRH.
↓
Increases circulating ACTH in fetus
↓
Hastens maturation of respiratory system
↓
So fetus picks the time to be born by increasing CRH secretion *(Pg. 451)*

18. From what type of cell was the karyotype in the following figure obtained?

A. Tumor cell
B. Spermatozoon
C. Ovum
D. Male autosome
E. Female autosome

Ans. (D)

Explanation:

Karyotyping of chromosomes: Chromosomes have been stained with **Giemsa's stain,** which produces typical **banding pattern.**

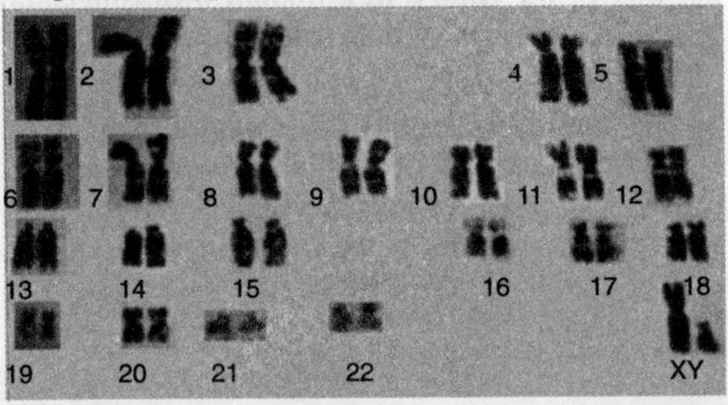

There are 46 chromosomes in males:
- 22 pairs of autosomes.
- X chromosome 2.
- Y chromosome.

Y chromosome is smaller than X chromosome.

(Pg. 412-413)

19. Size of the clitoris in a woman with congenital 17α-hydroxylase deficiency is:

A. Greater than size of the clitoris in a woman with congenital 21 β-hydroxylase deficiency
B. Same as size of the clitoris in a woman with congenital 21 β-hydroxylase deficiency
C. Less than size of the clitoris in a woman with congenital 21 β-hydroxylase deficiency

Ans. (C)

Explanation:

- 21 β-hydroxylase deficiency is common, accounting for 90% or more of enzyme deficiency cases.
- Production of **cortisol** and **aldosterone** is reduced so ACTH secretion and consequently production of precursor steroids are increased. These steroids are converted to androgens producing virilization.The characterstic pattern that develops in females in absence of treatment is the **adrenogenital syndrome.**

(Pg. 366, See also Ch. 20, Q. 13)

20. Size of the clitoris in a woman with congenital 11 β-hydroxylase deficiency is:

A. Greater than size of the clitoris in a woman with congenital 21 β-hydroxylase deficiency
B. Same as size of the clitoris in a woman with congenital 21 β-hydroxylase deficiency
C. Less than size of the clitoris in a woman with congenital 21 β-hydroxylase deficiency

Ans. (B)

Explanation:

In 11β-hydroxylase deficiency, virilization plus excess secretion of 11 deoxycortisol and 11 deoxycorticosterone takes place. Since former is active mineralocorticoid, patients with this syndrome also have salt and water retention and in 2/3 cases hypertension.

Treatment: Glucocorticoid treatment is indicated in all of the virilizing forms of congenital adrenal hyperplasia because it repairs glucocorticoid deficit and inhibits ACTH secretion, reducing abnormal secretion of androgens and other steroids.*(Pg. 366)*

21. Plasma LH concentration in a 59-year-old man is:

A. Greater than plasma LH concentration in a 59-year-old woman
B. Same as plasma LH concentration in a 59-year-old woman
C. Less than plasma LH concentration in a 59-year-old woman

Ans. (C)

22. hCG production in the first trimester of pregnancy is:

A. Greater than hCG production in the third trimester of pregnancy
B. Same as hCG production in third trimester of pregnancy
C. Less than hCG production in third trimester of pregnancy

Ans. (A)

Explanation:

hCG presence in urine in early pregnancy is the basis of various laboratory tests for pregnancy. *(Pg. 449)*

hCG secretion decreases after an initial marked rise.

23. hCS production in the first trimester of pregnancy is:

A. Greater than hCS production in the third trimester of pregnancy

B. Same as hCS production in the third trimester of pregnancy

C. Less than hCS production in the third trimester of pregnancy

Ans. (C)

Explanation:

- hCS (human chorionic somatomammotropin) is produced by syncytiotrophoblast cells.
- It has all the actions of GH (growth hormone) and apparently functions as **"maternal GH of pregnancy"** to bring about nitrogen, potassium, calcium retention, lipolysis and decreased glucose utilization.
- These actions divert glucose to fetus. The amount of hCS secreted is proportionate to the size of placenta and low hCS is **sign of placental insufficiency**. *(Pg. 450)*

UNIT IV. ENDOCRINOLOGY, METABOLISM AND REPRODUCTIVE FUNCTION

Chapter 24 Endocrine Functions of the Kidneys, Heart and Pineal Gland

1. **Renin is secreted by:**

   A. Cells in the macula densa
   B. Cells in the proximal tubules
   C. Cells in the distal tubules
   D. Juxtaglomerular cells
   E. Cells in the peritubular capillary bed

Ans. (D)

Explanation:

The **renin** in kidney extracts and the blood stream is produced by the juxtaglomerular cells (JG cells). *(Pg. 457)*

2. **Erythropoietin is secreted by:**

   A. Cells in the macula densa
   B. Cells in the proximal tubules
   C. Cells in the distal tubules
   D. Juxtaglomerular tubules
   E. Cells in the peritubular capillary bed

Ans. (E)

Explanation:

Erythropoietin is produced by interstitial cells in the peritubular capillary bed of the kidneys and by perivenous hepatocytes in the liver. *(Pg. 459)*

3. **Melatonin secretion would probably *not* be increased by:**

   A. Stimulation of the superior cervical ganglia
   B. Intravenous infusion of tryptophan
   C. Intravenous infusion of epinephrine
   D. Stimulation of the optic nerve
   E. Induction of pineal hydroxyindole-O-methyltransferase

Ans. (D)

Explanation:

Serotonin
↓ N-Acetyl transferase
N-Acetyl serotonin
↓ Hydroxy indole-O-methyl transferase
Melatonin ⟶ **secreted into blood**

(N-Acetyl transferase and Hydroxy indole-O-methyl transferase: **Pineal Parenchymal cells**)

Regulation of Secretion

Retinohypothalamic nerve fibers→Suprachiasmatic nuclei (Hypothalamus) → Intermediolateral gray Column of thoracic spinal cord→Preganglionic sympathetic neurons→superior cervical ganglion → Postganglionic neurons to pineal gland.

- Melatonin synthesis and secretion are increased during the dark period of the day and maintained at a low level during the daylight hours.
- This **diurnal variation** is brought about by norepinephrine (NE) secreted by the postganglionic sympathetic fibers that innervate the pineal gland.
- NE → acts in β adrenergic receptors → increases intracellular cAMP

↓

↑ increases N- acetyl transferase activity

↓

Increased melatonin synthesis and secretion

(Pg. 463)

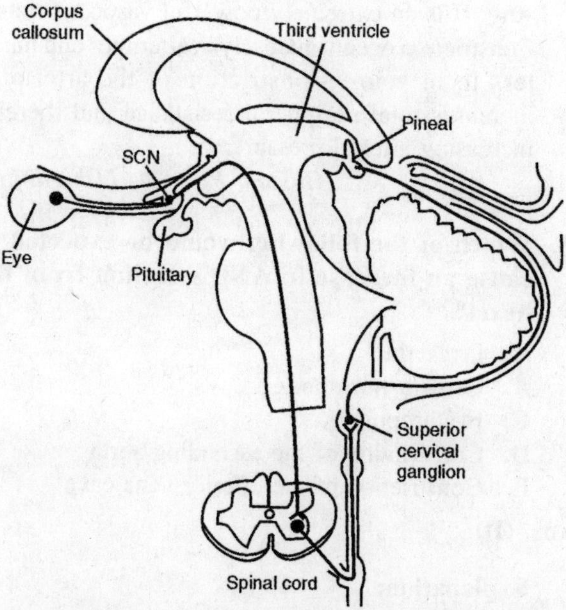

4. **When a woman who has been on a low-sodium diet for 8 days is given an intravenous injection of captopril, a drug that inhibits angiotensin-converting enzyme, one would expect:**
   A. Her blood pressure to rise because her cardiac output would fall
   B. Her blood pressure to rise because her peripheral resistance would fall
   C. Her blood pressure to fall because her cardiac output would fall
   D. Her blood pressure to fall because her peripheral resistance would fall
   E. Her plasma renin activity to fall because her circulating angiotensin I level would rise

Ans. (D)

Explanation:

Captopril and enalapril prevent conversion of Ang I to Ang II (Angiotensin-converting enzyme inhibitors/ACE inhibitors). *(Pg. 458)*

Ang. II is an extremely powerful vasoconstrictor. Constriction occurs intensely in arterioles and much less to in veins. Constriction of the arterioles increases total peripheral resistance and thereby increasing arterial pressure.

(Guyton, Pg. 224, 11th edition)

5. Which of the following would be expected to cause an increase in ANP secretion from the heart?

A. Prolactin
B. Growth hormone
C. Erythropoietin
D. Constriction of the ascending aorta
E. Constriction of the inferior vena cava

Ans. (D)

Explanation:

ANP secretion is increased when the ECF volume is increased by infusion of isotonic saline and when the atria are stretched. *(Pg. 461)*

6. Which of the following would *not* be expected to increase renin secretion?

A. Administration of a drug that blocks angiotesin-converting enzyme
B. Administration of a drug that blocks AT1 receptors
C. Administration of a drug that blocks β-adrenergic receptors
D. Constriction of the aorta between the celiac artery and the renal arteries
E. Administration of a drug that reduces ECF volume

Ans (C)

Explanation:

- Increased activity of sympathetic nervous system increases renin secretion.

- Increase is mediated by increased circulating catecholamines and by NE secreted by postganglionic renal sympathetic nerves.
- The catecholamines act mainly on β_1-adrenergic receptors on the JG cells and increases in renin are mediated by increase cAMP.

(Pg. 458)

Factors that affect renin secretion
Stimulatory
Increased sympathetic activity via renal nerves
Increased circulating catecholamines
Prostaglandins
Inhibitory
Increased Na^+ and Cl^- reabsorption across macula densa
Increased afferent arteriolar pressure
Angiotensin II
Vasopressin

7. Activation of receptors for ANP increases target cell:

A. cAMP
B. IP_3
C. Protein kinase A activity
D. Guanylyl cyclase activity
E. GTP

Ans. (D)

Explanation:

Natriuretic peptide receptors (NPR)

- Space cell membrane and have cytoplasmic domains that are guanylyl cyclases.
- Figure showing natriuretic peptide receptors. NPR-A and NPR-B have intracellular guanylyl cyclase domains while NPR-C has only small cytoplasmic domain.

(Pg. 461)

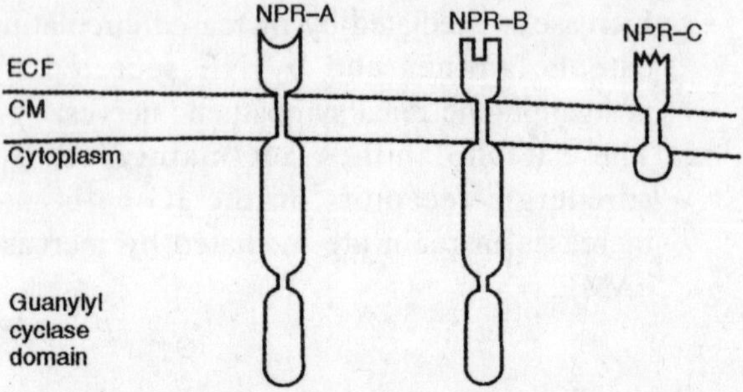

8. Erythropoietin:

A. Contains zinc
B. Contains iron
C. Is an important ligand for iron in the tissues
D. Stimulates renin secretion
E. Acts on red cell precursors in bone marrow

Ans. (E)

Explanation:

Erythropoietin increases the number of erythropoietin sensitive committed stem cells in bone marrow that are converted to RBC precursors and subsequently to mature RBC.

(Pg. 459)

9. Which of the following is *least* likely to contribute to the beneficial effects of angiotensin-converting enzyme inhibitors in the treatment of congestive heart failure?

A. Vasodilation
B. Decreased cardiac growth
C. Decreased cardiac afterload
D. Increased plasma renin activity
E. Decreased plasma aldosterone

Ans. (D)

Explanation:

Increased plasma renin activity → increases Ang II levels → which increases peripheral resistance → increasing arterial pressure. (See Ans. 4)

10. Which of the following is increased by infection of ACTH?

A. Thyroxine
B. Erythropoietin
C. Arginine vasopressin
D. Melatonin
E. Aldosterone

Ans. (E)

Explanation:

Hormone synthesis in zona glomerulosa

Cholesterol
↓ Block All
Pregnonolone
↓
Progesterone
↓
Deoxycorticosterone
↓ Aldosterone synthase
Corticosterone
↓ Aldosterone synthase
18 OH corticosterone
↓ Aldosterone synthase
Aldosterone

Chapter 25 Digestion and Absorption

1. The pathway from the intestinal lumen to the circulating blood for a short-chain fatty acid (< 10 carbon atoms) is:

A. Intestinal mucosal cell→chylomicrons→ lymphatic duct→systemic venous blood
B. Intestinal mucosal cell→hepatic portal vein blood→systemic venous blood
C. Space between mucosal cells→lymphatic duct →systemic venous blood
D. Space between mucosal cells → chylomicrons → lymphatic duct→systemic venous blood
E. Intestinal mucosal cell→LDL→hepatic portal vein blood→systemic venous blood

Ans. (B)

Explanation:

- The fate of FA in enterocyte depends on their size. FA containing less than 10-12 carbon atoms are water soluble enough that they pass through the enterocyte unmodified and are actively transported into the portal blood. They circulate as free FA (unesterified)
- FA containing > 10-12 carbon atoms are too insoluble for this. *(Pg. 475)*

2. Maximum absorption of short-chain fatty acids produced by bacteria occurs in the:

A. Stomach
B. Duodenum
C. Jejunum
D. Ileum
E. Colon

Ans. (E)

Explanation:

Short chain FA (SCFAs) are produced by colonic bacteria and are absorbed from colon. They are formed by the action of colonic bacteria on complex carbohydrates, resistant starches and other components of the dietary fiber. *(Pg. 475)*

3. Water is absorbed in the jejunum, ileum, and colon and excreted in the feces. Arrange these in order of the amount of water absorbed or excreted from greatest to smallest.

A. Colon, jejunum, ileum, feces
B. Feces, colon, ileum, jejunum
C. Jejunum, ileum, colon, feces
D. Colon, ileum, jejunum, feces
E. Feces, jejunum, ileum, colon

Ans. (C)

Explanation:

About 9 liters of fluid/day is presented to small intestine– 2 L from dietary sources, 7 L from GIT secretions, however only 1-2 L passes into the colon. *(Pg. 504)*

Total input =9000 ml

Reabsorbed

Jejunum	=	5500 ml
Ileum	=	2000 ml
Colon	=	1300 ml
		8800 ml

Balance in stool = 200 ml

4. Drugs and toxins that increase the cAMP content of the intestinal mucosa cause diarrhea because they:

A. Increase Na^{+}–K^{+} cotransport in the small intestine
B. Increase K^{+} secretion into the colon
C. Inhibit K^{+} absorption in the crypts of Lieberkiihn

D. Increase Na^+ absorption in the small intestine

E. Increase Cl^- secretion into the intestinal lumen

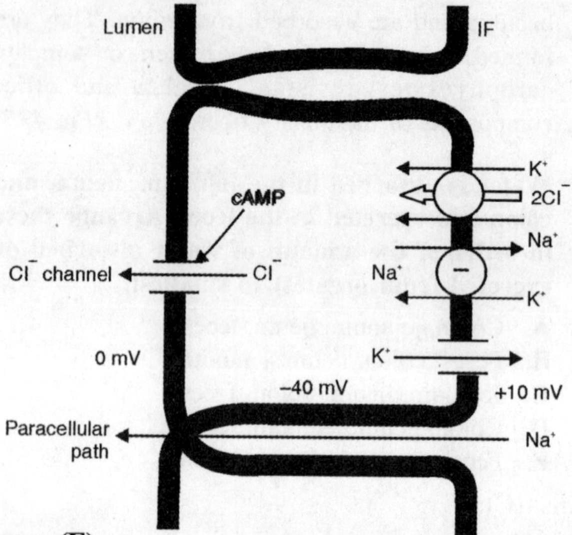

Ans. (E)

Explanation:

Figure showing movement of ions through enterocytes of small intestine.

- Cl^- normally enters enterocyte form the interstitial fluid via **Na^+-K^+-$2Cl^-$ co- transporters** in their basolateral membranes, and the Cl^- is then secreted into the intestinal lumen via channels that are regulated by various protein kinases (as shown in above figure).
- One of those is activated by **protein kinase A** and hence by cAMP.
- The cAMP concentration is increased in **cholera**.
- Cholera bacillus stays in the intestinal lumen but it produces a **toxin**, which causes prolonged activation of adenylyl cyclase and a marked increase in the intracellular cAMP concentration.
- In addition to increased Cl^- secretion, the function of the mucosal carrier for Na^+ is reduced, thus reducing NaCl absorption.

- The resultant increase in electrolyte and H_2O content of the intestinal contents causes the diarrhoea. *(Pg. 476)*

5. Which of the following are *incorrectly* paired?

A. Pancreartic α-amylase: starch
B. Elastase: tissues rich in elastin
C. Enteropeptidase: fatty acids
D. Renin: coagulated milk
E. Lingual lipase: digestion in the stomach

And. (E)

Explanation:

Enteropeptidases are the enzymes which are found in intestinal mucosa, They act on trypsinogen, leading to formation of trypsin.

$$\text{Trypsinogen} \xrightarrow{\text{Enteropeptidases}} \text{Trypsin}$$

6. Calcium absorption is increased by:

A. Hypercalcemia
B. Oxalates in the diet
C. Iron overload
D. 1, 25-dihydroxycholecalciferol
E. Increased Na^+ absorption

Ans. (D)

Explanation:

1, 25 $(OH)_2$ D_3 increases Ca^{+2} absorption from intestine by increasing formation of calbindin-D proteins. *(See also Chapter 21, Pg. 389)*

In questions 7-12 select:

A. If the item affects (a) below
B. If the item affects (b) below
C. If the item affects both (a) and (b), and
D. If the item affects neither (a) nor (b)
(a) Absorption of glucose
(b) Absorption of amino acids

7. Plasma K^+.

Ans. (D)

8. Na^+ in the intestinal lumen:

Ans. (C)

Explanation:

Glucose and AA transports require Na^+ because glucose and Na^+ share same cotransporter or symport, the sodium dependent glucose transporter (SGLT).

Similarly transport systems require Na^+ and co-transport aminoacids and Na^+ in a fashion similar to the cotransport of Na^+ and glucose.

(Pg. 470-472)

9. Plasma insulin:

Ans. (D)

Explanation:

Insulin does not affect glucose transport in intestine.

10. Phloridzin:

Ans. (A)

Explanation:

Glucose transport in the kidneys is inhibited as it is in intestine by a plant glycoside **Phloridzin**, which competes with d-glucose for binding to the carrier.

(Pg. 711)

11. Trypsin in intestinal lumen:

Ans. (B)

Explanation:

Trypsin is important for digestion of protein.

12. Ferritin in the intestinal mucosa:

Ans. (D)

Explanation:

Ferritin is storage form of Fe, not only in enterocytes, but also in many other cells.

(Pg. 477)

UNIT V. GASTROINTESTINAL FUNCTION

Chapter 26 Regulation of Gastrointestinal Function

Questions 1-4 refer to Figure below:

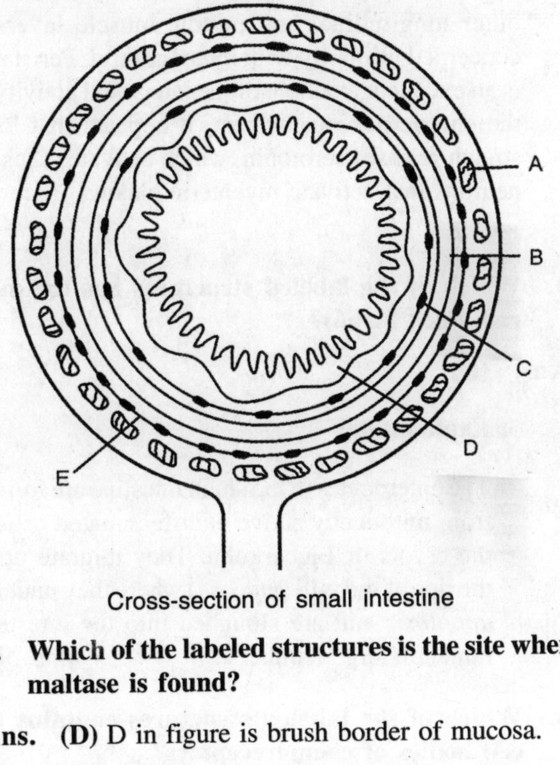

Cross-section of small intestine

1. Which of the labeled structures is the site where maltase is found?

Ans. (D) D in figure is brush border of mucosa.

Explanation:

The oligosaccharidases (Maltose, maltotriose, α- dextrins) responsible for the further digestion of the starch derivatives are located in the outer portion of the brush border, the membrane of the microvilli of the small intestine. *(Pg. 469)*

2. Which of the labeled structures is most concerned with integration of peristalsis?

Ans. (E)

Explanation:

Peristalsis is a reflex response that is initiated when the gutwall is stretched by the contents of the lumen and it occurs in all parts of GIT from the esophagus to rectum.

Myenteric plexus (Auerbach's plexus) between outer longitudinal and middle muscle layers is concerned primarily with motor control. Peristalsis is an excellent example of the integrated activity of the enteric nervous system. It appears that local stretch releases serotonin, which activates sensory neurons that activate myenteric plexus.

(Pg. 480)

3. Which of the labeled structures has the most rapid cell turnover?

Ans. (D)

Explanation:

The enterocytes in the small intestine are formed from mitotically active undifferentiated cells in the crypts of Lieberkuhn. They migrate up to the tips of the villi (*mucosa*) where they undergo *apoptosis* and are sloughed into the intestinal lumen in large numbers. *(Pg. 505)*

4. Which of the labeled structures contains the cell bodies of chemoreceptors?

Ans. (C) Submucous plexus (*Meissner's* plexus) between the middle circular layer and mucosa innervates the
- Glandular epithelium.
- Intestinal endocrine cells.
- Submucosal blood vessels

- It is primarily involved in the control of intestinal secretion. *(Pg. 479)*

Questions 5-8 refer to Table below:

Pattern	*Plasma bilirubin* *Direct*	*Indirect*	*Plasma alkaline phosphatase*	*Hematscocrit*	*Plasma bile acids*
A	—	—	—	—	↓
B	↑	↑↑	—	—	—
C	↑↑	↑	↑	—	↓
D	↑	↑↑	—	↓	—
E	↑	↑↑	↑	—	↑

– = no change; ↑ = increase; ↑↑ = marked increase; ↓ = decrease

5. Which set of data would be found in a patient with a gallstone obstructing the common bile duct?

Ans. (C)

Explanation:

Conjugation will be normal, so high levels of direct bilirubin (conjugated bilirubin).

6. Which set of data would be found in a patient with intravascular hemolysis?

Ans. (D)

Explanation:

High levels of unconjugated (Indirect bilirubin).

7. Which set of data would be found in a patient with infectious hepatitis?

Ans. (B)

Explanation:

No conjugation in liver, so high levels of indirect bilirubin, while direct bilirubin will fall. Hematocrit remains same.

8. Which set of data would be found in a patient with a resection of the ileum?

Ans. (A)

Explanation:

Enterohepatic circulation of bile acids will be affected. So bile acids will be decreased.

9. **Removal of the entire colon would be expected to cause:**
   - **A.** Death
   - **B.** Megaloblastic anemia
   - **C.** Severe malnutrition
   - **D.** An increase in the blood level of ammonia in patients with cirrhosis of the liver
   - **E.** Decreased urinary urobilinogen

Ans. (D)

Explanation:

Vitamin B_{12} deficiency can be produced by diseases of *distal ileum* leading to megaloblastic anaemia. Large amounts of NH_3 are formed by the deamination process and additional amounts are continually formed in the gut by bacteria and then absorbed in the blood. Therefore if liver does not form urea its plasma concentration rises rapidly resulting in coma and death.

10. **In infants, defecation often follows a meal. The cause of colonic contractions in this situation is:**
    - **A.** The gastroileal reflex
    - **B.** Increased circulating levels of CCK
    - **C.** The gastrocolic reflex
    - **D.** Increased circulating levels of somatostatin
    - **E.** The enterogastric reflex

Ans. (C)

Explanation:

Distention of the stomach by food initiates contractions of the rectum and frequently a desire to defecate. The response is called the **gastrocolic reflex**, although there is some evidence that it is due to an action of **gastrin** on the colon and is not neurally mediated. Because of the response, defecation after meals is the rule in children. In adults, habit and cultural factors play a large role in determining when defecation occurs. *(Pg. 511)*

11. After a meal rich in carbohydrates is ingested, insulin secretion is probably stimulated by:

A. GLP-1 (7-36) amide
B. CCK
C. Serotonin
D. VIP
E. Gastrin

Ans. (A)

Explanation:

Glucagon-like polypeptide (GLP-1) acts as additional gut factor that stimulates insulin secretion. *(Pg. 347, 487)*

12. The symptoms of the dumping syndrome (discomfort after meals in patients with intestinal short circuits such as anastomosis of the jejunum to the stomach) are caused in part by:

A. Increased blood pressure
B. Increased secretion of glucagon
C. Increased secretion of CCK
D. Hypoglycemia
E. Hyperglycemia

Ans. (D)

Explanation:

Because of rapid absorption of glucose from intestine and resultant hyperglycemia leading to abrupt rise in insulin secretion, gastrectomized patients sometimes develop hypoglycemic symptoms about 2 hours after meals. *(Pg. 496)*

13. Which of the following has the highest pH?

A. Gastric juice
B. Bile in the gallbladder
C. Pancreatic juice
D. Saliva
E. Secretions of the intestinal glands

Ans. (C)

Explanation:

Hepatic Duct	**Gallbladder Bile**
Bile pH 7.8-8.6	7.0-7.4

So in gallbladder, acidification of bile occurs. *(Pg. 503)*

Pancreatic juice is alkaline pH= 8.0. *(Pg. 497)*

14. After complete hepatectomy, a rise would be expected in the blood level of:

A. Glucose
B. Fibrinogen
C. 25-hydroxycholecalciferol
D. Conjugated bilirubin
E. Estrogens

Ans. (E)

Explanation:

Plasma levels of:
- Glucose
- Fibrinogen

falls because

- Gluconeogenesis occurs in liver.
- Synthesis of plasma proteins in liver.
- 25 (OH) D_3 falls because
  25 hydroxylase enzyme that converts
  Vit D_3
  ↓ 25 hydroxylase (found in liver)
  25 OH D_3 (Cholecalciferol)

So no conversion, so level falls.

- Conjugation of bilirubin occurs in liver, so hepatectomy leads to lower levels.

- **Estrogens-hepatic** metabolism of estrogens to inactive metabolites occurs in liver, so in hepatectomy, estrogen levels rise. *(Pg. 440)*

15. Which of the following would not be produced by total pancreatectomy?

A. Vitamin E deficiency
B. Hyperglycemia
C. Metabolic acidosis
D. Weight gain
E. Decreased absorption of amino acids

Ans. (D)

Explanation:

- Removal of endocrine pancreas → leads to hyperglycaemia (no insulin) → so associated with **weight loss.**
- Metabolic acidosis (no insulin).
- Removal of exocrine pancreas → leads to decreased absorption of AA (no digestion of protein, no enzymes).

Chapter 27 Circulating Body Fluids

In questions 1-5, match the immunoglobulin in each question with the lateral characteristic that are most associated with it. Each lettered characteristic may be selected once, more than once, not at all:

A. Complement fixation
B. Secretory immunity
C. Release of histamine from basophils and mast cells
D. Tetramer
E. Antigen recognition by B cells

1. IgA
Ans. (B)
2. IgD
Ans. (E)
3. IgE
Ans. (C)
4. IgG
Ans. (A)
5. IgM
Ans. (A)

Explanation:

Immunoglobulin	*Function*
1. IgG	Complement activation
2. IgA	Localized protection in external secretions (tears, intestinal secretions etc.)
3. IgM	Complement activation
4. IgD	Antigen recognition by B cells
5. IgE	1. Reagin activity 2. Releases histamine from basophils and mast cells

All immunoglobulins are mainly monomer, except IgD which exists as tetramer.

(Pg. 529)

Questions 6-9 refer to figure below:

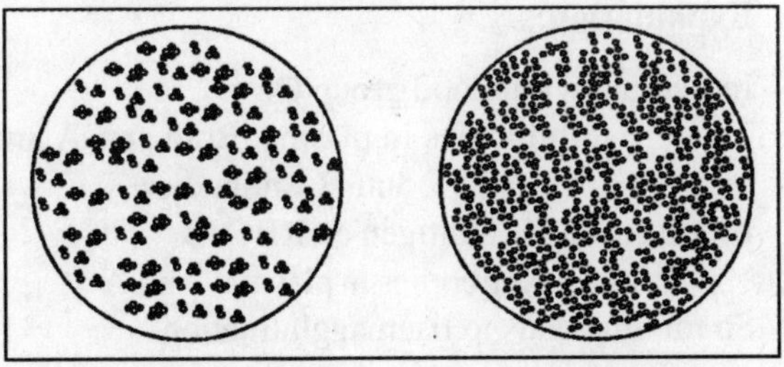

A B

Red blood cells in plasma

6. Which of the patterns indicates a mismatch if red cells from a donor are mixed plasma from a recipient?

Ans. (A)

Explanation:

When recipients plasma has agglutinins against the donors RBC, the cells agglutinate and hemolyze. Free hemoglobin is liberated into the plasma leading to jaundice and renal tubular damage.

(Pg. 538)

7. Which of the patterns would be seen if plasma from an individual with blood type B were mixed with red cells from an individual with blood type O?

Ans. (B)

Explanation:

Plasma of person with blood group B has anti-A antibodies while RBC of person with blood group O has neither A nor B antigens, so no agglutination.

8. Which of the patterns would be seen if plasma from an individual with blood type O were mixed with red cells from an individual with blood type B?

Ans. (A)

Explanation:

Individual with blood group O:

Antibodies in plasma: Both anti-A and anti-B Antibodies.

Blood group B : Antigen on RBC: B

Antibodies in plasma: Anti A

So mixing leads to haemagglutination.

9. In which of the patterns would the hemoglobin in the plasma be highest?

Ans. (A)

Explanation:

Haemagglutination leads to hemolysis of RBC. Free haemoglobin is released in circulation.

10. Which of the following is *not* primarily a function of blood plasma?

A. Transport of hormones
B. Maintenance of red cell size
C. Transport of chylomicrons
D. Transport of antibodies
E. Transport of O_2

Ans. (E)

Explanation:

Transport of gases is function of haemoglobin which is red, oxygen carrying pigment in the red blood cells (RBCs). *(Pg. 534)*

11. A hematocrit of 41% means that in the sample of blood analyzed: *(Refer to earlier Figure)*

A. 41% of the hemoglobin is in the plasma
B. 41% of the total blood volume is made up of blood plasma
C. 41% of the total blood volume is made up of red and white blood cells and platelets

D. 41% of the hemoglobin is in red blood cells
E. 41% of the formed elements in blood are red blood cells

Ans. (C)

Explanation:

Hematocrit or packed cell volume (PCV) is the most accurate and simplest of all tests in clinical hematology for detecting the presence and degree of anemia or polycythemia.

- The % of blood that is cells is called hematocrit.
- So PCV of **41%** means 41% of total blood volume is made up of RBC, WBC and platelets, and remainder is plasma.
- It is measured in a centrifuge machine, using wintrobe tube (hematocrit tube).
- These values vary tremendously depending on whether the person has anaemia, on degree of body activity and on altitude.

(Guyton, 11th Ed., Pg. 169)

12. In normal human blood:

A. The eosinophil is the most common type of white blood cell
B. There are more lymphocytes than neurophils
C. The iron is mostly in hemoglobin
D. There are more white cells than red cells
E. There are more platelets than red cells

Ans. (C)

Explanation:

Hemoglobin a globular molecule, made up of 4 subunits. Each subunit contains a **heme** moiety conjugated to a polypeptide. Heme is an iron containing porphyrin derivative. *(Pg. 534)*
Normal RBC counts: 5.4 million/cmm^3 of blood (males)= 4.8 millon/cmm^3 of blood (Females)
Total WBC count: 4000-11000/cmm^3 of blood

Granulocytes

Neutrophils	:	are 50-70% of total WBC
Eosinophils	:	1-4% of total WBC
Basophils	:	0.4% of total WBC

Agranulocytes

Lymphocytes	:	20-40% of total WBC
Monocytes	:	2-8% of total WBC

13. Lymphocytes:

A. All originate from the bone marrow after birth
B. Are unaffected by hormones
C. Convert to monocytes in response to antigens
D. Interact with eosinophils to produce platelets
E. Are part of the body's defense against cancer

Ans. (E)

Explanation:

Lymphocytes specially T lymphocytes, mediates cellular immunity and defend against tumors.

(Pg. 525)

14. Production of the type of cell shown in figure 27.2 is increased by:

A. Interleukin-2 (IL-2)
B. Granulocyte colony-stimulating factor (G-CSF)
C. Erythropoietin
D. Interleukin-4 (IL-4)
E. Interleukin-5 (IL-5)

Ans. (B)

Explanation:

G-CSF acts on granulocytes and is produced by endothelial cells, fibroblasts and monocytes.

(Pg. 520)

15. The cell shown in figure below probably does *not* contain:

A. Actin
B. Free radicals

C. Myeloperoxidase
D. Cathepsins
E. A Y chromosome

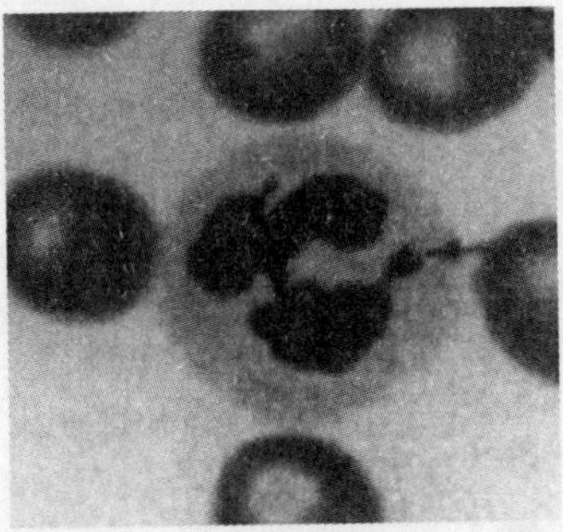

Diagram showing drumstick (arrow) in WBC

Ans. **(E)**

Explanation:

Soon after cell division, has started during embryonic development, one or the other of the two X chromosomes of the somatic cells in normal females becomes functionally inactive. However, the details of the inactivation process are still incompletely understood. The choice of which X chromosome remains active is random, so normally one X chromosome remains active in approximately half of cells and other X chromosome is active in other half. In normal cells, the inactive X chromosome condenses and can be seen in various types of cells, usually near the nuclear membrane, as the **Barr body body/sex chromatin**. The inactive X chromosome is also visible as small 'drumstick' of chromatin projecting from the nuclei of 1-15% of the polymorphonuclear leukocytes in females, but not in males. *(Pg. 412)*

16. In which of the following diseases is the structure of the hemoglobins that are produced normal but their amount reduced?

A. Chronic blood loss
B. Sickle cell anemia

C. Hemolytic anemia
D. Thalassemia
E. Transfusion reactions

Ans. (D)

Explanation:

- Chains are normal in structure.
- Decreased amounts/absent because of defects in the regulatory portion of the globin genes. The α and β thalassemias are defined by decreased or absent α and β polypeptides respectively. *(Pg. 535)*

Sickle cell anaemia: Abnormal hemoglobin (HbS) polymerizes at low O_2 tensions and this causes RBC to become sickle shaped, hemolyze and form aggregates that block blood vessels. The result is severe hemolytic anaemia knowm as sickle cell anaemia.

Dangerous hemolytic transfusion reaction: Occurs when blood is transfused into an individual with an incompatible blood type. Free hemoglobin is liberated into the plasma due to agglutination and hemolysis. *(Guyton, 11th Ed, Pg. 426)*

Chronic blood loss leads to micocytic hypochromic anaemia, RBC that are then produced are much smaller than normal and have too little hemoglobin inside them.

17. Which of the following plasma proteins is *not* synthesized primarily in the liver?

A. Angiotensinogen
B. C-reactive protein
C. Angiotensin II converting enzyme
D. α_2- Macroglobulin
E. Fibrinogen

Ans. (C)

Explanation:

Angiotensin II converting enzyme (ACE) is an ectoenzyme that exists in 2 forms:

Somatic form

- Found throughout the body.

Germinal form

- Post meiotic spermatogenic cells and spermatozoa. *(Pg. 455)*

18. Cells responsible for innate immunity are activated most commonly by:

A. Glucocorticoids
B. Pollen
C. Carbohydrate sequences in bacterial cell walls
D. Eosinophils
E. Cytoplasmic proteins of bacteria

Ans. **(C)**

Explanation:

The cells that mediate innate immunity are:

1. Neutrophils.
2. Macrophages.
3. Natural killer (NK) cells.
   - All these cells respond to lipid and carbohydrate sequences unique to bacterial cell walls and to other substances characteristic of tumor and transplant cells. In addition, some bacteria cause release of uric acid from damaged tissues and uric acid crystals activates immune system.
   - The **activated cells** produce their effects via complement and other systems. Their cytokines also activate cells of the acquired immune system. *(Pg. 524)*

19. Number of light chains in a basic immunoglobulin molecule is:

A. Greater than the number of heavy chains in a basic immunoglobulin molecule
B. Same as the number of heavy chains in a basic immunoglobulin molecule
C. Less than the number of heavy chains in a basic immunoglobulin molecule

Ans: (B)

Explanation:

The basic component of each Ig is a symmetric unit containing 4 polypeptide chains.The 2 long chains are called **heavy chains,** whereas the two short chains are called **light chains.** *(Pg. 529)*

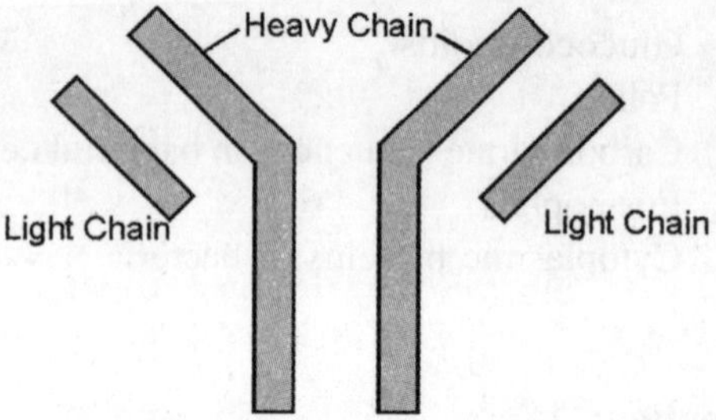

Immunoglobin Molecule

20. Amount of CD4 glycoprotein on surface of helper T cell is:

A. Greater than the amount of CD4 glycoprotein on surface of cytotoxic T cell

B. Same as the amount of CD4 glycoprotein on surface of cytotoxic T cell

C. Less than the amount of CD4 glycoprotein on surface of cytotoxic T cell

Ans. (A)

Explanation:

The **MHC** protein (Major histocompatibility complex) peptide complexes on the surface of antigen presenting cells (APC) bind to appropriate T cells. Therefore, receptors on T cells must recognize a very wide variety of complexes.

- CD8 occurs on the surface of cytotoxic T cells that bind MHC-I protiens.
- CD4 occurs on the surface of helper T cells that bind MHC II protein.
- Activated CD8 cytotoxic T cells kills targets directly while activated CD4 helper T cells secrete cytokines that activate other lymphocytes. *(Pg. 527)*

Chapter 28 Origin of the Heart-beat and the Electrical Activity of the Heart

Questions 1-4 refer to the following Figure:

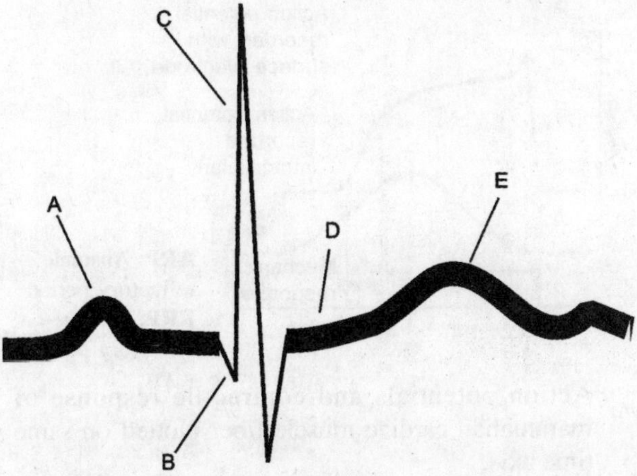

E.C.G.

1. Which of the labels identifies the part of the ECG that corresponds to ventricular repolarization?

Ans. (E)

Explanation:

Ventricular repolarization is suggested by E-wave.

(Pg. 550-551)

2. Which of the labels identifies the Q wave?

Ans. (B)

3. Which of the labels identifies the part of the ECG that corresponds to maximum opening of ventricular Na^+ channels?

Ans. (C)

4. Which of the labels identifies the part of the ECG that corresponds to maximum opening of ventricular Ca^{2+} channels?

Ans. (D)

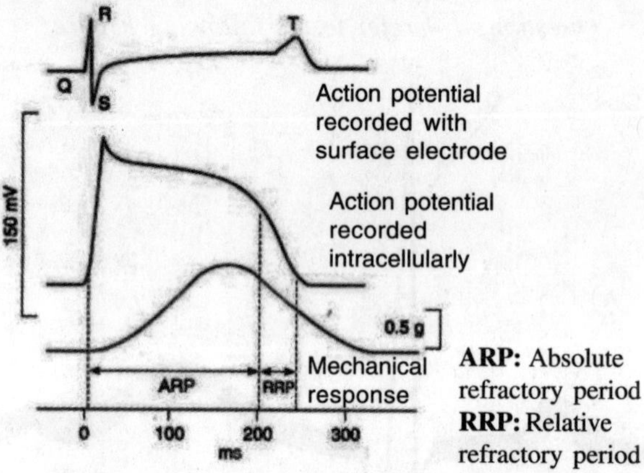

Action potentials and contractile response of mammalian cardiac muscle fiber plotted on same time axis.

Explanation:

Waves of E.C.G.

P wave is produced by atrial depolarization (action potential of ventricular muscle).

QRS duration is produced by ventricular depolarization and atrial repolarization.

QT interval is produced by ventricular depolarization plus ventricular repolarization.

ST interval is produced by ventricular repolarization.

- AP and ECG are plotted on the same time axis but with zero points on the vertical scale.
- The transmembrane AP of single cardiac muscle cells is characterized by:
  1. Rapid depolarization (Due to Na^+ influx through Na^+ channels).
  2. Plateau (Ca^{+2} influx through slowly opening Ca^{+2} channels).
  3. Slow repolarization (net K^+ efflux through multiple types of K^+ channels). *(Pg. 548)*

5. Which of the following normally has the most prominent prepotential?

A. Sinoatrial node
B. Atrial muscle cells
C. Bundle of His
D. Purkinje fibers
E. Ventricular muscle cells

Ans. (A)

Explanation:

Rhythmically discharging cells have a membrane potential that after each impulse, declines to the firing level. Thus this prepotential or pacemaker potential triggers the next impulse.

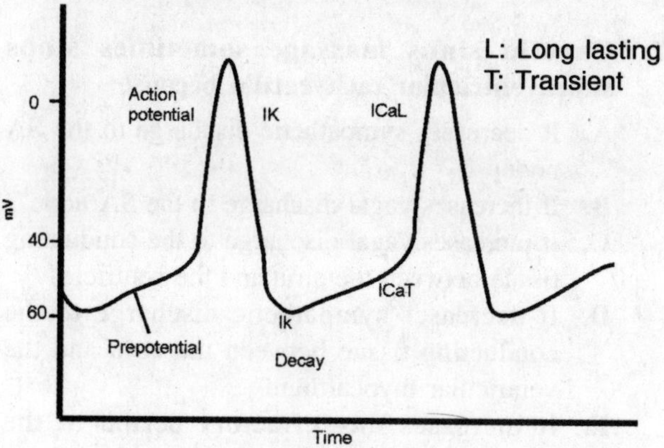

- At the peak of each impulse, IK then begins and brings about repolarization. IK then declines and as K^+ efflux decreases, the membrane begins to depolarize, forming 1st part of the prepotential. Ca^{+2} channels then open and complete the prepotential.
- The AP in SA and AV nodes are largely due to Ca^{+2} with no contribution by Na^+ influx. **Prepotentials** are **prominent** only in SA and AV nodes. However "latent pacemakers" are present in other portions of conduction system that can take over when SA and AV nodes are depressed or conduction from them is blocked. *(Pg. 548)*

6. In second-degree heart block:

A. The ventricular rate is lower than the atrial rate
B. The ventricular ECG complexes are distorted
C. There is a high incidence of ventricular tachycardia
D. Stroke volume is decreased
E. Cardiac output is increased

Ans. (A)

Explanation:

In 2nd degree heart block, not all atrial impulses are conducted to the ventricles, e.g., a ventricular beat may follow every second or every third atrial beat (2:1 block, 3:1 block etc).

7. Carotid sinus massage sometimes stops supraventricular tachycardia because:

A. It decreases sympathetic discharge to the SA node
B. It increases vagal discharge to the SA node
C. It increases vagal discharge to the conducting tissue between the atria and the ventricles
D. It decreases sympathetic discharge to the conducting tissue between the atria and the ventricular myocardium
E. It increases the refractory period of the ventricular myocardium

Ans. (C)

Explanation:

Atrial/A-V nodal paroxysmal tachycardia, both of which are called supraventricular tachycardias, usually occurs in young, otherwise healthy people and they generally grow out of the predisposition to tachycardia after adolescence. In general supraventricular tachycardia frightens a person tremendously and may cause weakness during paroxysm, but only seldom does permanent harm come from the attack.

(Guyton, 11th edition, Pg. 152)

8. **Currents caused by opening of which of the following channels contribute to the repolarization phase of the action potential of ventricular muscle fibers?**

A. Na^+ channels
B. Cl^- channels
C. Ca^{2+} channels
D. K^+ channels
E. HCO_3^- channels

Ans. (D)

Explanation:

Repolarization is due to net K^+ efflux through multiple types of K^+ channels.

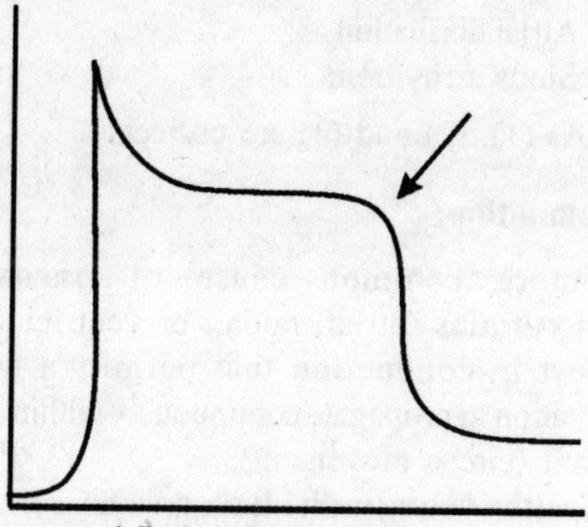

A.P of venticular muscle

In questions 9-11, one or more than one of the answers may be correct. Select:

A. If (1), (2) and (3) are correct
B. If (1) and (3) are correct
C. If (2) and (4) are correct
D. If only (4) is correct
E. If all are correct

9. **In complete heart block:**

1. Fainting may occur because the atria are unable to pump blood into the ventricles
2. Ventricular fibrillation is common

3. The atrial rate is lower than the ventricular rate
4. Fainting may occur because of prolonged periods during which the ventricles fail to contract

Ans. **(D)**

Explanation:

When conduction from atria to ventricles is completely interrupted, complete (3rd degree) heart block results and ventricles beat at a low rate (idioventricular rhythm) independent of atria.

10. Reentry is a common cause of:

1. Paroxysmal artial tachycardia
2. Paroxysmal nodal tachycardia
3. Atrial fibrillation
4. Sinus arrhythmia

Ans. (A) (1), (2) and (3) are correct

Explanation:

A more common cause of **paroxysmal arrhythmias** (atrial, nodal, or ventricular) is a defect in conduction that permits a wave of excitation to propagate continuously within a closed circuit (circus movement). *(Pg. 536)*

In **healthy young individuals** breathing at a normal rate, the heart rate varies with the phases of **respiration,** it accelerates during inspiration and decreases during expiration, especially if the depth of breathing is increased. This is called **sinus arrhythmia,** a normal phenomenon. *(Pg. 554)*

11. In a patient with the long QT syndrome, one might find:

1. A gain-of-function mutation in a cardiac Na^+ channel
2. Abnormal endolymph in the middle ear
3. A loss-of-function mutation in the HERG gene
4. An ankyrin abnormality

Ans. (E) All are correct

Explanation:

Long QT syndrome

- QT interval is prolonged.
- Cardiac repolarization is irregular.
- Incidence of ventricular arrhythmia is more.

Cause:

- Different drugs.
- Electrolyte abnormalities.
- Myocardial ischemia.
- Congenital.

Congenital:

- Mutation of genes.
- Reduced function of various K^+ channels by alterations in their structure.

It is of 2 forms:

One form	Other form
Inhibits K^+ channel by reducing the amount of ankycin isoform that links it to cytoskeleton	Increases function of cardiac Na^+ channel

(Pg. 558)

12. Height of T waves when the plasma K^+ level is 5.5 meq/L is:

A. Greater than the height of T waves when the plasma K^+ is 8.5 meq/L

B. Same as the height of T waves when the plasma K^+ is 8.5 meq/L

C. Less than the height of T waves when the plasma K^+ is 8.5 meq/L

Ans. (C)

Explanation:

As plasma K^+ level rises, the first change in ECG is appearance of tall peaked T waves, a manifestation of altered repolarization. At higher K^+ levels, paralysis of atria and prolongation of QRS complexes occur. *(Pg. 563)*

13. In normal adults, height of the R wave in lead V1 of the ECG is:

A. Greater than the height of R wave in lead V_5 of the ECG

B. Same as the height of R wave in lead V_5 of the ECG

C. Less than the height of R wave in lead V_5 of the ECG

Ans. (C)

Explanation:

There are six unipolar chest leads (precordial leads) designated V_1-V_6 *(Pg. 551)*

- In leads V_1 and V_2 - the QRS recordings of normal are mainly negative because chest electrode in these leads is near the base of heart that to apex and base of heart is the direction of electronegativity during most of ventricular depolarization process. Conversely, QRS complexes in lead V_4, V_5 and V_6 are mainly positive because chest electrode in these leads is near apex of heart which is direction of electropositivity during most depolarization. *(Guyton, 11th Ed, Pg. 129)*

14. Interval between an atrial premature beat and the next normal beat is:

A. Greater than the interval between ventricular premature beat and the next normal beat

B. Same as the interval between a ventricular premature beat and the next normal beat

C. Less than the interval between a ventricular premature beat and the next normal beat

Ans. (C)

Explanation:

Premature beats that originate in an ectopic ventricular focus usually have bizarre shaped prolonged QRS complexes because of slow spread of impulse from focus through ventricular muscle to rest of ventricle.

- Usually incapable of exciting the bundle of His.
- In mean time, next succeeding normal SA nodal impulse depolarizes the atria.
- P wave is usually buried in QRS of extrasystole.
- If normal impulse reaches ventricles, they are still in refractory period following depolarization from ectopic focus.
- 2nd impulse from SA node produces a normal beat because ventricular premature beats are followed by a **compensatory pause** that is usually longer than the pause after an atrial extrasystole.
- Further ventricular premature beats do not interrupt regular discharge of SA node, whereas atrial premature beats often interrupt and reset normal rhythm. *(Pg. 558)*

15. Slope of prepotential in SA node after stimulation of vagus is:

A. Greater than the slope of prepotential in SA node after stimulation of sympathetic nerves to heart

B. Same as the slope of prepotential in SA node after stimulation of sympathetic nerves to heart

C. Less than the slope of prepotential in SA node after stimulation of sympathetic nerves to heart

Ans. **(C)**

When cholinergic vagus fibers to nodal tissue are stimulated, membrane becomes hyperpolarized and slope of prepotential is decreased, therefore acetylcholine released at nerve endings increases K^+ conductance of nodal tissue.

While stimulation of sympathetic cardiac nerves makes membrane potential fall more rapidly and rate of spontaneous discharge increases, therefore, NE released at sympathetic endings facilitates opening of Ca^{+2} channels, increasing Ca^{+2} influx and rapidity of depolarization phase of impulse.

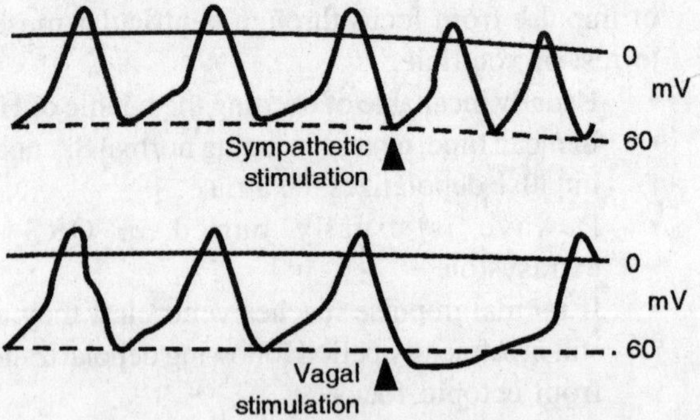

Figure showing effect of sympathetic and vagus stimulation on membrane potential of SA node

Chapter 29 The Heart as a Pump

Questions 1-5 refer to Figure 29.1. Select the letter in the figure that identifies the following:

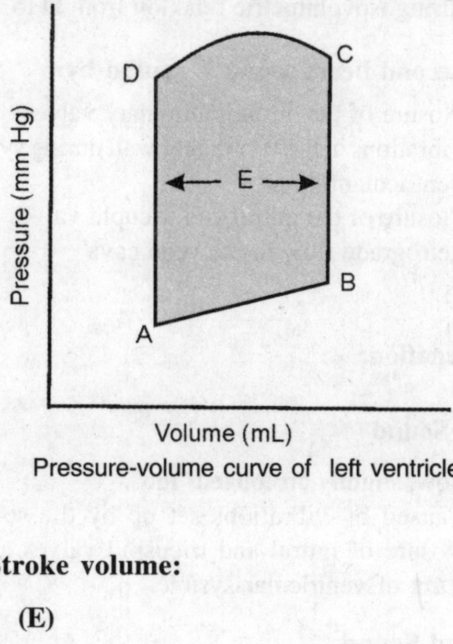

Pressure-volume curve of left ventricle

1. Stroke volume:

Ans. (E)

2. Point where aortic valve opens:

Ans. (C)

3. Point where aortic valve closes:

Ans. (D)

4. Point where mitral valve opens:

Ans. (A)

5. Point where mitral valve closes:

Ans. (B)

Explanation:

1. During diastole: Ventricle fills and pressure increases from A to B.
2. Pressure then rises sharply from B to C during isovolumetric contraction and from C to D.
3. At D, aortic valve closes and pressure falls during isovolumetric relaxion from D to A.

6. The second heart sound is caused by:

A. Closure of the aortic pulmonary valves
B. Vibrations in the ventricular wall during systole
C. Ventricular filling
D. Closure of the mitral and tricupid valves
E. Retrograde flow in the vena cava

Ans. (A)

Explanation:

First Sound

- Low, slightly prolonged "lub".
- Caused by vibrations set up by the sudden closure of mitral and tricuspid valves at the **start** of ventricular systole.

Second Sound

- Shorter.
- High pitched "dup"
- Caused by vibrations associations with closure of the aortic and pulmonary valves just after the **end** of ventricular systole.

(Pg. 569)

7. The fourth heart sound is caused by:

A. Closure of the aortic and pulmonary valves
B. Vibrations in the ventricular wall during systole
C. Ventricular filling
D. Closure of the mitral and tricuspid valves
E. Retrograde flow in the vena cava

Ans. (C)

Explanation:

Third Sound

- Slow, low pitched.
- Coincides with the period of rapid ventricular filling and is due to vibrations set up by the inrush of blood.

Fourth Sound

- Due to ventricular filling and is rarely heard in normal adults. *(Pg. 569)*

8. **The dicrotic notch on the aortic pressure curve is caused by:**

   A. Closure of the mitral valve
   B. Closure of the tricuspid valve
   C. Closure of the aortic valve
   D. Closure of the pulmonary valve
   E. Rapid filling of the left ventricle

Ans. **(C)**

Explanation:

- The dicrotic notch, a small oscillation on the falling phase of the pulse wave caused by vibrations set up when the arctic valve snaps shut.
- It is visible if pressure wave is recorded but is not palpable at wrist.
- The pulmonary artery pressure curve also has a dicrotic notch produced by closure of the pulmonary valves *(Pg. 568)*

9. **During exercise, a man consumes 1.8 L of oxygen per minute. His arterial O_2 content is 190 mL/L, and the O_2 content of his mixed venous blood is 134 mL/L. His cardiac output is approximately:**

   A. 3.2 L/min
   B. 16 L/min

C. 32 L/min
D. 54 L/min
E. 160 mL/min

Ans. (C)

Explanation:

$$CO = \frac{O_2 \text{ consumption}}{[AO_2] - [VO_2]}$$
$$= \frac{18 \text{ L/L (180 mL/L/min)}}{(190 - 134)}$$
$$= \frac{180}{56}$$
$$= 32 \text{ L/min}$$

10. The work performed by the left ventricle is substantially greater than that performed by the right ventricle, because in the left ventricle:

A. The contraction is slower
B. The wall is thicker
C. The stroke volume is greater
D. The preload is greater
E. The afterload is greater

Ans. (E)

Explanation:

- Ventricular work/beat correlates with O_2 consumption.
- Work = Stroke volume × Mean arterial pressure in pulmonary artery (for RV)/ aorta (LV).
- Since aortic pressure is 7 times greater than pulmonary artery pressure, stroke work of LV approximately 7 times the stroke work of RV.
- In theory 25% increase in stroke volume without change in arterial pressure should produce the same increase in O_2 consumption as 25% increase in arterial pressure without change in smoke volume. However for unknown reasons, pressure work produces a greater increase in O_2 consumption then volume work.

- So increase in **afterload causes a greater increase** in cardiac O_2 **consumption then an increase** in preload does. *(Pg. 575)*

11. Starling's law of the heart:

A. Does not operate in the failing heart
B. Does not operate during exercise
C. Explains the increase in heart rate produced by exercise
D. Explains the increase in cardiac output that occurs when venous return is increased
E. Explains the increase in cardiac output when the sympathetic nerves supplying the heart are stimulated

Ans. (D)

Explanation:

- According to **Starling law of heart or Frank Starling law.**
- Energy of contraction is directly proportional to the initial length of cardiac muscle fiber.
- For heart, the length of muscle fibers (extent of preload) is proportionate to the end diastolic volume (Venous return). *(Pg. 572)*

In questions 12-15, match the item in each question with lettered abnormality that is most closely associated with it. Each lettered abnormality may be selected once, more than once or not at all.

A. Aortic stenosis
B. Aortic insufficiency
C. Mitral stenosis
D. Patent ductus arteriosus
E. Pulmonary hypertension

12. Bounding corrigan pulse:

Ans. (B) Aortic insufficiency

Explanation:

When aortic valve is incompetent, the pulse is

particularly strong and force of systolic ejection may be sufficient to make head nod with each heart beat. The pulse is called collapsing corrigan or water hammer pulse.

(A water hammer is a evacuated glass tube ½ filled with water that was a popular toy, when held in hand and inverted, it delivers a short, hard knock).

(Pg. 568)

13. Loud, snapping 2nd heart sound:

Ans. (E) Pulmonary hypertension

14. Diastolic murmur loudest over the apex of the heart:

Ans. (C) Mitral stenosis

Explanation:

- Murmurs due to mitral disease are usually heard at the apex of heart.
- When orifice is narrow, stenosis, blood flow through it in normal direction is accelerated and turbulent. *(Pg. 570)*

15. Decreased perfusion of coronary arteries

Ans. (A) Aortic stenosis

Explanation:

Blood flow to the left ventricle is decreased in patients with stenotic aortic valves because in aortic stenosis the pressure in the left ventricle must be higher than that in aorta to eject the blood. Consequently, the coronary vessels are severely compressed during systole. Patients with this disease are particularly prone to develop symtoms of myocardial ischemia, in part because of this compression and in part because the myocardium requires more O_2 to expel blood through the stenotic aortic valve.

(Pg. 621)

Chapter 30 Dynamics of Blood and Lymph Flow

1. Which of the following has the highest *total* cross-sectional area in the body?

A. Arteries
B. Arterioles
C. Capillaries
D. Venules
E. Veins

Ans. (C)

Explanation:

Vessel	Cross-sectional area (cm^2)
1. Aorta	2.5
2. Small arteries	20
3. Arterioles	40
4. Capillaries	2500
5. Venules	250
6. Small veins	80
7. Venae cavae	8

(Guyton, 11th Ed, Pg. 162, 578)

2. Lymph flow from the foot is:

A. Increased when an individual rises from the supine to the standing position
B. Increased by massaging the foot
C. Increased when capillary permeability is decreased
D. Decreased when the valves of the leg veins are incompetent
E. Decreased by exercise

Ans. (B)

Explanation:

The flow in lymph vessels is massaged by muscle contractions of the organs and contraction of arterioles and venules, with which they are associated.

- Flow in collecting lymphatics is further aided by movements of skeletal muscle (main factor).
- Negative intrathoracic pressure during inspiration.
- Suction effect of high velocity flow of blood in the veins in which the lymphatics terminate.
- Various agents increase lymph flow (lymphagogues) by increasing capillary permeability.
- Agents that cause contraction of **smooth** muscle also increase lymph flow from the intestine. *(Pg. 593)*

3. The pressure in a capillary in skeletal muscle is 35 mm Hg at the anterior end and 14 mm Hg at the venular end. The interstitial pressure is 0 mm Hg. The colloid osmotic pressure is 25 mm Hg in the capillary and 1 mm Hg in the interstitium. The net force producing fluid movement across the capillary wall at its arteriolar end is:

A. 3 mm Hg out of the capillary
B. 3 mm Hg into the capillary
C. 10 mm Hg out of the capillary
D. 11 mm Hg out of the capillary
E. 11 mm Hg into the capillary

Ans. (D)

Explanation:

(Guyton, 11th Ed, Pg. 189) Starling forces

Forces tending to more fluid outward		mmHg.
1.	Capillary pressure (arterial end)	35
2.	Interstitial fluid colloid osmotic pressure	1
	Total	= 36
Forces tending to move fluid inward		
1.	Capillary colloid osmotic pressure	25
2.	Interstitial hydrostatic pressure	0
	Total	= 25
Therefore summation of forces		
	Outward	36
	Inward	25
Net outward force (at arterial end)		11

4. Which of the following does *not* occur as blood passes through the systemic capillary?

A. Its hematocrit increases
B. Its hemoglobin dissociation curve shifts to the left
C. Its protein content increases
D. Its pH decreases
E. Its red blood cells increase in size

Ans. (B)

Explanation:

As the blood passes through capillaries, RBC become thimble or parachute shaped, with the flow pushing the center ahead of the edges, due to pressure in center of the vessel.

- Structure of wall of capillary is composed of single layer of endothelial cells. The structure of walls varies from organ to organ. In many beds, including those in skeletal, cardiac and smooth muscle, the junctions between endothelial cells permit passage of molecules upto 10 mm in diameter. It also appears that plasma and its dissolved proteins are taken up by endocytosis, transported across endothelial cells and discharged by exocytosis (Vesicular transport). *(Pg. 577)*
- Due to gaseous exchange across capillary, when CO_2 enters, pH falls. *(Pg. 592)*

5. The velocity of blood flow:

A. Is higher in the capillaries than the arterioles
B. Is higher in the veins than in the venules
C. Is higher in the veins than the arteries
D. Falls to zero in the descending aorta during diastole
E. Is reduced in a constricted area of a blood vessel

Ans. (B)

Explanation:

Velocity (V) = Flow (Q) /Area of conduit (A)
The average velocity of fluid movement at any point in a system of tubes in parallel is inversely proportional to the total cross-sectional area at that point.

Venules - Total cross-sectional area 250 cm^2
Veins - Total cross-sectional area 80 cm^2

So in veins velocity of flow is more than venules.

(Pg. 584)

6. **When the radius of the resistance vessels is increased, which of the following is increased?**
   - **A.** Systolic blood pressure
   - **B.** Diastolic blood pressure
   - **C.** Viscosity of the blood
   - **D.** Hematocrit
   - **E.** Capillary blood flow

Ans. (E)

Explanation:

Relation between flow in a long narrow tube, viscosity of fluid and radius of tube is expressed by *Poiscuille-Hagan formula*

$$F = (P_A - P_B) \times \frac{\pi}{8} \times \frac{1}{\eta} \times \frac{r^4}{L}$$

F = Flow
P_A- P_B = Pressure difference between two ends
η = Viscosity
r = Radius of tube
L = Length of tube

Since $F = \frac{P_A - P_B}{R}$

Therefore $R = \frac{8\,\eta L}{\pi\, r^4}$

- Therefore flow varies directly and resistance inversely with fourth power of radius.

- Flow is doubled by increase of only 19% in its radius.
- Blood flow and resistance in vivo are markedly affected by small changes in caliber of vessels.

(Pg. 584)

7. When the viscosity of the blood is increased, which of the following is increased?

A. Mean blood pressure
B. Radius of the resistance vessels
C. Radius of the capacitance vessels
D. Central venous pressure
E. Capillary blood flow

Ans. (A)

Explanation:

Resistance to blood flow is determined not only by radius of blood vessels but also by viscosity of blood. *(Pg. 585)*

8. A pharmacologist discovers a drug that stimulates the production of VEGF receptors. He is excited because his drug might be of value in the treatment of:

A. Coronary artery disease
B. Cancer
C. Emphysema
D. Diabetes insipidus
E. Dysmenorrhea

Ans. (A)

Explanation:

Many factors are involved in angiogenesis. A key compound is the protein growth factor vascular endothelial growth factor (VEGF). It appears to be primarily responsible for vasculogenesis.

(Pg. 581)

9. Why is the dilator response to injected acetylcholine changed to a constrictor response when the endothelium is damaged?

A. More Na^+ is generated
B. More bradykinin is generated
C. The damage lowers the pH of the remaining layers of the artery
D. The damage augments the production of endothelin by the endothelium
E. The damage interferes with the production of No by the endothelium

Ans. (E)

Explanation:

- Acetylcholine
- Bradykinin
- VIP
- Shear stress

} Act on endothelium to cause release of No
↓
NO causes relaxation of vascular smooth muscle

while

- Adenosine
- ANP
- H_2 receptors

} Relaxation of vascular smooth muscle that is independent of endothelium

(Pg. 598)

10. Sildenafil (Viagra) has seen extensive use in aiding the production of erections in man. However, it can also produce transient inability to distinguish between blue and green. This is because it:

A. Dilates arteries in the penis and the retina
B. Produces selective constriction of arteries in the penis and the retina
C. Reduces the concentration of cGMP in the penis and the retina
D. Inhibits the production of endothelin in the penis and the retina
E. Inhibits the phosphodiesterases found in the penis and the retina

Ans. (E)

Explanation:

Erection is mediated by efferent parasympathetic fibers that are present in pelvic splanchnic nerves (Nervi erigentes) and contain acetylcholine and VIP. There are also nonadrenergic noncholinergic fibers in the nervi erigentes and these contain large amounts of **NO synthase** the enzyme that catalyzes formation of NO.

NO activates cyclase

↓

Guanylyl cyclase → GTP → cGMP leading to smooth muscle relaxation.

So NO plays an important role in the erection.

Sildenafil (Viagra) inhibits breakdown of cGMP by phosphodiesterases, so is used in treatment of impotence.

- A type of phosphodiesterase is found in retina and **Sildenafil** also produces significant inhibition of this phosphodiesterase. So one of side effects of this drug is transient loss of ability to discriminate between blue and green. *(Pg. 428)*

In questions 11-14, which of the labelled structures in the following Figure:

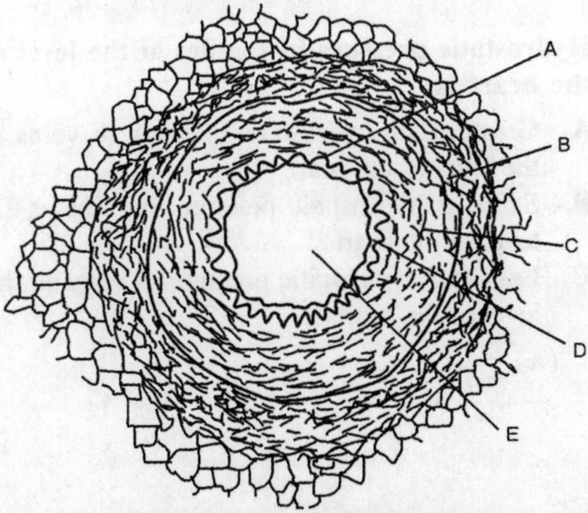

Cross-section of small artery

11. Is the site of the initial visible lesion in athero-sclerosis?

Ans. (D)

Explanation:

Initial visible site of lesion in atherosclerosis is endothelium.

Flowing blood creates a force on the endothelium that is parallel to long axis of vessel. This shear stress (stretch) produce marked changes in expression of genes in the endothelial cells that are related to cardiovascular function.

(Pg. 583)

12. Is reduced in size in the presence of angiotensin II:

Ans. (E) Lumen

13. Is responsible for maintaining blood flow during diastole:

Ans. (A) Intima

14. Responds to shear stress via receptors respon-sive to stretch:

Ans. (D) Endothelium

15. Hydrostatic pressure in venules at the level of the heart is:

A. Greater than hydrostatic pressure in veins at the level of the heart

B. Same as hydrostatic pressure in veins at the level of the heart

C. Less than hydrostatic pressure in veins at the level of the heart

Ans. (A)

16. Permeability of capillaries in the lungs is:

A. Greater than the permeability of capillaries in the liver

B. Same as permeability of capillaries in the liver

C. Less than the permeability of capillaries in the liver

Ans. (C)

Explanation:

In liver, clefts between capillary endothelium cells are wide open, so all dissolved substances of plasma, including plasma proteins can pass from blood into liver tissues.

(Guyton, 11th Ed., Pg. 182)

Chapter 31 Cardiovascular Regulatory Mechanisms

1. **Which of the following is *incorrectly* paired?**
   - **A.** Angiotensin-converting enzyme: kinin metabolism
   - **B.** Stimulation of the vagus nerve in the neck: bradycardia
   - **C.** Prostacyclin: vasodilatation
   - **D.** Increased pressure in the cartiod sinuses: decreased sympathetic discharge to arterioles
   - **E.** Increased H^+ in tissues: vasoconstriction in tissues

Ans. (E)

Explanation:

The metabolic changes that produce vasodilation include (in most tissues):

- Decrease in O_2 tension.
- Decrease in pH.
- Increase in CO_2 tension.
- Increase in osmolality.

Cause: Relaxation of arterioles and precapillary sphincters. The direct dialator action of CO_2 is most pronounced in skin and brain.

- ACE (angiotensin converting enzyme) inactivates bradykinin so interferes with kinin metabolism.

(Pg. 444, 445)

2. **When a pheochromocytoma (tumor of the adrenal medulla) suddenly discharges a large amount of epinephrine into the circulation, the patient's heart would be expected to:**
   - **A.** Increase because the increase in blood pressure stimulates the carotid and aortic baroreceptors
   - **B.** Increase because epinephrine has a direct chronotropic effect on the heart

C. Increase because of increased tonic parasympathetic discharge to the heart
D. Decrease because the increase in blood pressure stimulates the carotid and aortic chemoreceptors
E. Decrease because of increased tonic parasympathetic discharge to the heart

Ans. (B)

Explanation:

Most adrenal medullary tumors (pheochromocytoma) secrete NE or epinephrine, or both and produce sustained hypertension. Epinephrine produces tachycardia when plasma level is about twice the resting value. *(Pg. 360)*

3. Vasopressin secretion is increased by:

A. Increased pressure in the right ventricle
B. Decreased pressure in the right ventricle
C. Increased pressure in the right atrium
D. Decreased pressure in the right atrium
E. Increased pressure in the aorta

Ans. (D)

Explanation:

- ECF volume also affects vasopressin secretion.
- If ECF volume is low vasopressin secretion is increased.
- If ECF volume is high vasopressin secretion is decreased.
- There is an inverse relationship between the rate of vasopressin secretion and the rate of discharge in afferents from stretch receptors in low and high pressure portions of the vascular system.

Low pressure receptors are in:

- Great vein.
- Right and left atria.
- Pulmonary vessels.

High pressure receptors:

- Carotid sinus.
- Aortic arch. *(Pg. 245)*

Low pressure receptors monitor fullness of vascular system. Low pressure receptors are main mediators for vasopressin secretion.

4. Catecholamines acting on α-adrenergic receptors:

A. Increase the contractility of cardiac muscle
B. Increase the rate of discharge of the sinoatrial node
C. Increase cardiac output
D. Constrict coronary arteries by a direct action on these blood vessels
E. Dilate blood vessels in skeletal muscle

Ans. (D)

Explanation:

Catecholamines act via α_1 and α_2 receptors on coronary blood vessels to produce constriction and via β_2 receptors to cause dilation. *(Pg. 227)*

5. Which of the following would be expected to raise blood pressure?

A. Prostacyclin
B. A drug that inhibits angiotensin-converting enzyme
C. A drug that inhibits NO synthase
D. A drug that inhibits V_{1A} vasopressin receptors
E. A drug that inhibits endothelin activity

Ans. (C)

Explanation:

Endothelium-derived relaxing factor (NO) acts on endothelial cells and play a key role in vasodilation.

Many of the vasoactive substances produced by endothelial cells are also produced by other cells and have different functions in other parts of the body. In questions 6-10, select:

A. If the item is associated with (a) below
B. If the item is associated with (b) below
C. If the item is associated with both (a) and (b)
(a) Endothelin-1
(b) NO
D. If the item is associated with neither (a) nor (b)

6. Brain:

Ans. (C)

Explanation:

NO is synthesized from arginine in a reaction catalyzed by **nitric oxide synthase (NOS)** 3 isoforms are these:
NOS 1 is found in nervous system.
NOS 2 is found in macrophages and other immune cells.
NOS 3 is found in endothelial cells:

- NO is important for brain function. Unlike other transmitters, it is gas, which crosses cell membranes with ease and binds directly to guanyl cyclase. It may be the signal by which postsynaptic neurons communicate with presynaptic endings in LTP (Long-term potentiation) and LTD (Long-term depression). *(Pg. 115)*
- Endothelial cells produce endothelin-1, one of the most potent vasoconstrictor agents yet isolated. It is found in brain and kidneys as well as endothelial cells. *(Pg. 600)*

7. Intestine:

Ans. (B)

Explanation:

In GIT, NO is a major dilator of smooth muscle.
(Pg. 599)

8. Kidneys:

Ans. (C)

Explanation:

- A possible mediator is NO, in the renin secretion from juxtaglomerular cells, but the identity of the signal remains unsettled. *(Pg. 458)*
- Endothelin-1 is also found in kidneys. *(Pg. 600)*

9. Lungs:

Ans. (B)

Explanation:

Epithelium of paranasal sinuses appears to produce NO which is bacteriostatic and helps prevent infections. *(Pg. 664)*

10. Immune cells:

Ans. (B)

Explanation:

NO is necessary for the cytotoxic activity of macrophages, including their ability to kill cancer cells. *(Pg. 599)*

In questions 11-16, match the vasoactive compound in each question with the lettered mechanism of action that is most closely associated with it. Each lettered item may be selected once, more than once, or not at all.

A. Activates guanylyl cyclase
B. Activates protein kinase A
C. Activates phospholipase C
D. Activates phospholipase A_2
E. Activates tyrosine kinase

11. Angiotenstin II

Ans. (C)

12. Endothelin-1:

Ans. (D)

13. Nitric oxide:

Ans. (A)

14. Bradykinin:

Ans. (C)

15. VIP:

Ans. (B)

16. Substance P:

Ans. (C)

Explanation:

AT_1 (angiotensin II receptors) are serpentine receptors coupled by a G protein to phospholipase C and angiotensin II increases cytostolic Ca^{+2} level. *(Pg. 457)*

Bradykinin is a vasodilator acts via G proteins. **Substance P** also acts as vasodilator and also increases capillary permeability. This local neural mechanism is called the **axon reflex** when substance P is released from nerve endings. **Endothelin-1** is a potent vasoconstrictor, which acts via G proteins. The concentration of endothelin-1 is elevated in congestive heart failure and after myocardial infarction (MI), so it may play a role in the pathophysiolorsy of these diseases. *(Pg. 600)*

VIP is a vasodilator, causes dilation of peripheral blood vessels.

17. Which of the vasoactive compounds listed above (11-16) cause vasoconstriction in vivo?

Ans. 11, 12 (Angiotenstin II; Endothelin-1)

18. Which of the vasoactive compounds (11-16) cause vasodilatation in vivo?

Ans. 13, 14, 15, 16 *(Pg. 603)*

Explanation:

Summary of factors affecting the caliber of arterioles:

Constriction	*Dilation*
a. Endothelial products	
• Endothelin-1	NO
• Locally released platelet serotonin	Kinins
• Thromboxane A_2	Prostacyclin
b. Circulating hormones	
• Epinephrine (Except in skeletal muscle and liver)	Epinephrine in skeletal muscle and liver
• NE	CGRPα
• AVP	Substance P
• Angiotensin II	Histamine
• Neuropeptide Y	ANP
	VIP

Chapter 32 Circulation Through Special Regions

In questions 1-13, select the single best answer. Questions 1-5 refer to Figure.

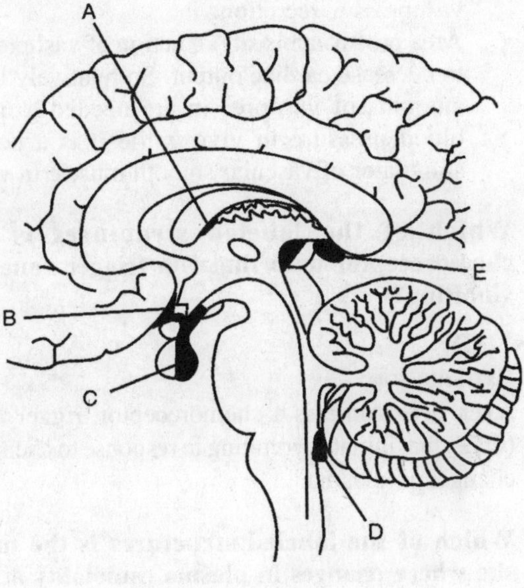

Sagittal view of the human brain

1. Which of the labeled structures is the main site at which hypothalamic hormones leave the brain?

Ans. (C)

Explanation:

'Neuro-hemel organs' (post pituitary), i.e., areas in which polypeptides secreted by neurons enter the circulation, e.g., oxytocin and vasopressin.

2. Which of the labeled structures is the main site at which vasopressin acts to decrease cardiac output?

Ans. (B)

Explanation:

- OVLT is site of osmoreceptor controlling vasopressin secretion.
- Area prostroma is site of action of vasopressin to decrease cardiac output. So relatively large amounts of vasopressin are needed to raise blood pressure in vivo while it is a potent stimulator of vascular smooth muscle in vitro.

3. Which of the labeled structures is the chemoreceptor area that is a trigger zone for vomiting?

Ans. (D)

Explanation:

Area prostroma is a chemoreceptor trigger zone (CTZ) that initiates vomiting in response to chemical changes in plasma.

4. Which of the labeled structures is the main site where changes in plasma osmolality act to alter vasopressin secretion?

Ans. (B)

Explanation:

- OVLT is site of osmoreceptor controlling vasopressin secretion.
- Area prostroma is site of action of vasopressin to decrease cardiac output. So relatively large amounts of vasopressin are needed to raise blood pressure in vivo while it is a potent stimulator of vascular smooth muscle in vitro.

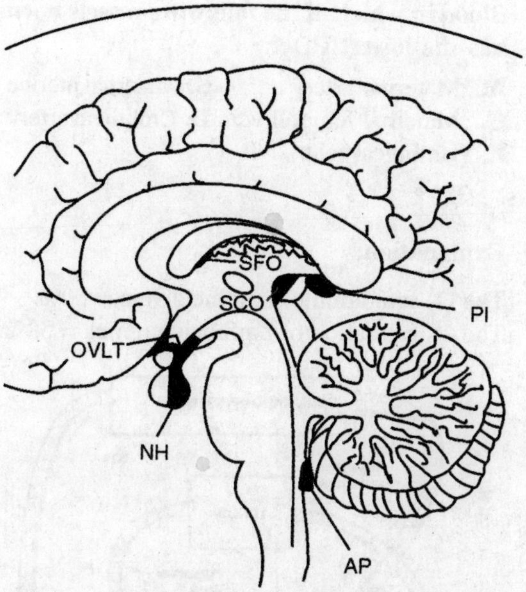

Circumventricular organs

5. **Which of the labeled structures is the main site at which angiotensin II acts to increase water intake?**

Ans. (A)

Explanation:

Angiotensin II acts on subfornical organ and possibly on SFO to increase water intake.
Circumventricular organs includes:

1. Post pituitary and adjacent part of median eminence of hypothalamus.
2. Area prostroma.
3. The organum vasculosum of the lamina terminalis (OVLT, Supraoptic crest).
4. Subfornical organ (SFO).

All have fenestrated capillaries and because of their permeability they are said to be "outside-blood brain barrier".

6. Blood in which of the following vessels normally has the lowest PO_2?

A. Maternal artery
B. Maternal uterine vein
C. Maternal femoral vein
D. Umbilical artery
E. Umbilical vein

Ans. (D)

Explanation:

The O_2 saturation of umbilical vein = 80%.
The O_2 saturation of umbilical arteries = 58%.

(Pg. 628)

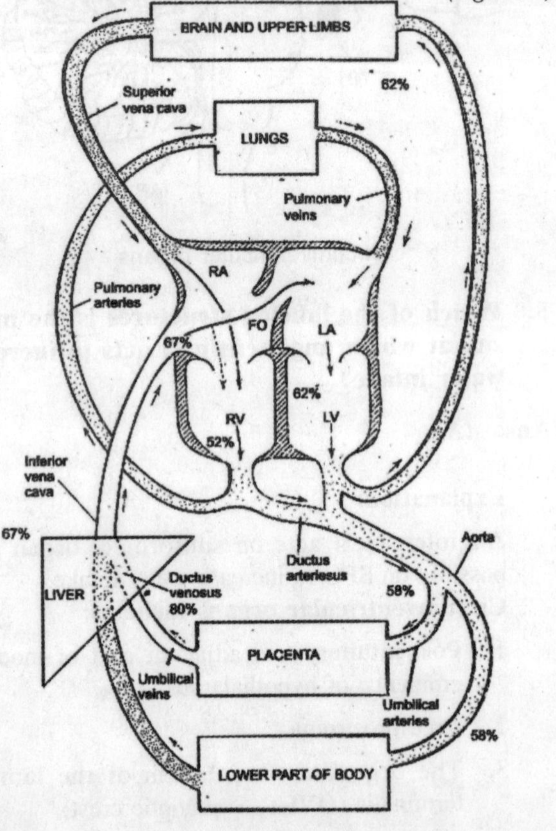

Scheme of the fetal circulation. The degree of deoxygenation is shown by the intensity of shading. RA=right atrium; LA=left atrium; RV=right ventricle; LV=left ventricle; FO=foraman ovale; P=pulmonary trunk; A= arota.
% of saturation of blood flowing in the indicated blood vessel.

Fetal Circulation

- Fetal lungs are inactive and fetus depends completely on the placenta for O_2 and nutrient supply.
- Oxygenated fetal blood from the placenta passes through the umbilical vein to the liver.
- Approximately ½ of blood from the placenta passes through the liver and remainder bypasses the liver and reaches the IVC (Inferior vena cava) through ductus venosus.
- In IVC, blood from ductus venosus joins the blood returning from the lower trunk and extremities. This combined stream in turn merges with the blood from the liver through the hepatic veins.
- The large stream of blood that passes through foramen ovale into left atrium is joined by blood returning from the lungs and it is pumped out by the left ventricle into aorta.
- Fetal blood that leaves placenta is 80% saturated but the saturation of blood that passes through foramen ovale is reduced to 67% (because of mixing with desaturated blood returning from lower part of body and liver).
- Addition of desaturated blood from lungs reduces the O_2 saturation of left ventricular blood to 62% which is the level of saturation of blood reaching the head and upper extremities.
- The blood in RV which is a mixture of desaturated superior vena caval blood, coronary venous blood and inferior vena caval blood is only 52% saturated.
- When the major portion of this blood traverses the ductus arteriosus, and joins that pumped out by the left ventricle, the resulting O_2 saturation of the blood travelling to the lower part of body and back to placenta is 58%.

(Berne and Levy Physiology, 5th Ed, Pg. 429)

7. The pressure differential between the heart and the aorta is least in the:

A. Left ventricle during systole
B. Left ventricle during diastole
C. Right ventricle during systole
D. Right ventricle during diastole
E. Left atrium during systole

Ans. (A)

Explanation:

Pressure (mm Hg)				*Pressure differential (mm Hg) between aorta and*	
	Aorta	LV	RV	LV	RV
Systole	120	121	25	- 1	95
Diastole	80	0	0	80	80

(Pg. 621)

8. Injection of tissue plasminogen activator (t-PA) would probably be most beneficial.

A. After at least 1 year of uncomplicated recovery following occlusion of a coronary artery
B. After at least 2 months of rest and recuperation following occlusion of a coronary artery
C. During the second week after occlusion of a coronary artery
D. During the second day after occlusion of a coronary artery
E. During the second hour after occlusion of a coronary artery

Ans. (E)

Explanation:

t-PA must be given early in the course of a stroke to be of maximum benefit and this is why stroke has become a condition in which rapid diagnosis and treatment have become important. *(Pg. 620)*

9. Which of the following organs has the greatest blood flow per 100 g of tissue?

A. Brain
B. Heart muscle

C. Skin
D. Liver
E. Kidneys

Ans. (E) Kidneys

Explanation:

	Blood flow ml/100 g/min	
Kidneys	**420**	1260
Heart	**84**	250
Liver	**57**	1500
So highest blood flow/ml/100 g/min = Kidneys.		
So highest blood flow/ ml/min = Liver.		

(Pg. 612)

10. Which of the following organs has the most permeable capillaries?

A. Brain
B. Posterior pituitary gland
C. Liver
D. Small intestine
E. Kidneys

Ans. (C)

Explanation:

In most

- Endocrine glands
- Intestinal villi
- Parts of kidneys
- Cytoplasm of endothelial cells

} is attenuated to form gaps called **Fenestrations** (20-100 nm D)

In liver:

- Sinusoidal capillaries extremely porus.
- Endotheluim is **discontinuous.**
- Gaps occur between endothelial cells that are closed by membranes.

- Some of gaps are (600 nm in diameter and others may be as large as 3000 nm in diameter).

(Pg. 578)

11. Which of the following does *not* dilate arterioles in the skin?

A. Increased body temperature
B. Epinephrine
C. Bradykinin
D. Substance P
E. Vasopressin

Ans. **(E)**

Explanation:

- Vasopressin is a potent vasoconstrictor.
- Rest all are vasodilators.

12. A baby boy is brought to the hospital because of convulsions. In the course of a workup, his body temperature and plasma glucose are found to be normal, but his cerebrospinal fluid glucose is 12 mg/dL (normal, 65 mg/dL). A possible explanation of his condition is:

A. Constitutive activation of GLUT 3 in neurons
B. SGLT 1 deficiency in astrocytes
C. GLUT 5 deficiency in cerebral capillaries
D. GLUT 1 55 K deficiency in cerebral capillaries
E. GLUT 1 45 K deficiency in microglia

Ans. (D)

Explanation:

Glucose is the major ultimate source of energy for nerve cells. Its passive penetration of blood-brain barrier is slow, but it is transported across the walls of brain capillaries by glucose transporter (GLUT-1). The brain contains 2 forms of GLUT-1, (GLUT-1 55k) and (GLUT-1 45k). GLUT-1 55k is present in high concentration in brain capillaries. Infants with **congenital GLUT-1** deficiency develop low **CSF glucose concentrations** in the presence of normal **plasma glucose** and they have seizures and **delayed development.**

(Pg. 615)

13. Recently, there has been great interest in the role of inflammation in the production of atherosclerosis. Evidence for this includes:

A. Chronic low-grade fever
B. Increased proliferation of the intima in the medium-sized and small arteries
C. High cholesterol contents of intestinal bacteria
D. Possible examples of molecular mimicry
E. Premature rupture of atherosclerotic plaques

Ans. (D)

Explanation:

There has been a correlation between circulating antibodies to **chlamydia pneumoniae** and atherosclerotic plaques. This micro organism has an amino acid sequence in its plasma membrane that resembles a sequence in heart α myosin heavy chains and injection of this sequence causes autoimmune inflammation and fibrosis of coronary arteries in mice, an example of **molecular mimicry.**

(Pg. 623)

14. Amount of water transported into cerebrospinal fluid is:

A. Greater than the amount of water transported out of the cerebrospinal fluid
B. Same as the amount of water transported out of the cerebrospinal fluid
C. Less than the amount of water transported out of the cerebrospinal fluid

Ans. (B)

Explanation:

Lumbar CSF pressure is normally 70-180 mm CSF. At pressure of 112 mm CSF, which is the average normal CSF pressure, filtration and absorption are equal. Below a pressure of approximately 68 mm CSF, absorption stops. *(Pg. 613)*

15. Blood flow in the endocardial portion of the myocardium during systole is:

A. Greater than the blood flow in the epicardial portion of the myocardium during systole
B. Same as the blood flow in the epicardial portion of the myocardium during systole
C. Less than the blood flow in the epicardial portion of myocardium during systole

Ans. (C)

Explanation:

Heart like skeletal muscle, compresses its blood vessels when it contracts. The pressure inside the left ventricle is slightly higher than in aorta during systole. Consequently flow occurs in the arteries supplying endocardial portion of left ventricle only during diastole, although the force is sufficiently dissipated in the more superficial portions of the left ventricular myocardium to permit some flow in this region throughout the cardiac cycle. Because there is no blood flow during systole in the subendocardial portion of left ventricle, this portion more prone to ischemia and most common site of myocardial infarction. *(Pg. 621)*

16. Amount of blood brought to the liver by the hepatic artery is:

A. Greater than the amount of blood brought to the liver by the portal vein
B. Same as the amount of blood brought to the liver by the portal vein
C. Less than the amount of blood brought to the liver by the portal vein

Ans. (C)

Explanation:

Hepatic blood is derived from 2 sources:

- Portal vein (3/4 of blood flow).
- Hepatic artery (1/4 of blood flow).

Portal vein provides 3/4 of blood flow because portal vein has already passed through gastrointestinal capillary bed, much of O_2 of portal vein blood flow has already been extracted. The hepatic artery delivers the remaining ¼ of blood, which is fully saturated with O_2. Hence about 3/4th of O_2 used by the liver is derived from hepatic arterial blood.

(Berne and Levy Physiology, 5th Ed, Pg. 428)

Chapter 33 Cardiovascular Homeostasis in Health and Disease

In questions 1-13, select the single best answer. Each of the patients in questions 1-5 has a blood pressure of 85/40 mm Hg. Match the condition in each question with the emergency treatment that is most appropriate. Each lettered treatment may be selected once, more than once, or not at all.

A. Injection of dopamine
B. Infusion of concentrated human albumin
C. Infusion of isotonic saline solution
D. Injection of epinephrine
E. Infusion of whole blood

1. Girl stung by a bee:

Ans. (D)

Explanation:

In anaphylactic shock, **epinephrine** has a highly beneficial and almost specific effect that must represent more than just constriction of the dilated vessels. *(Pg. 641)*

2. Man bleeding from a stab wound:

Ans. (E)

Explanation:

In hemorrhagic, traumatic and surgical shock, the primary cause of the shock is blood loss, so the treatment should include early and rapid transfusion of adequate amounts of compatible whole blood.

3. Woman burned over 35% of her body in a kitchen fire:

Ans. (B)

Explanation:

In shock due to burns and other conditions in which there is hemoconcentration, plasma is the treatment of choice to restore the fundamental defect, i.e., the loss of plasma. 'Plasma expanders', i.e., solution of sugars of high molecular weight and related substances that do not cross capillary walls have some merit. Concentrated human serum albumin and other hypertonic solutions expand the blood volume by drawing fluid out of the interstitial spaces. They are valuable in emergency treatment but have the disadvantage of further dehydrating the tissues of an already dehydrated patient.

4. Woman who had a myocardial infarction 24 hours previously:

Ans. (A)

Explanation:

Because dopamine produces:

- Renal **vasodilation** and has positively ionotropic effect while producing vasoconstriction elsewhere, dopamine is of value in the treatment of traumatic and cardiogenic shock. *(Pg. 361)*

5. Man with severe diarrhea:

Ans. (C)

6. Plasma renin activity is most likely to be lower than normal:

A. In congestive heart failure
B. In hemorrhagic shock
C. In shock due to infection with gram-negative bacteria
D. In essential hypertension
E. During quiet standing

Ans. (D)

7. **From your knowledge of physiology, which of the following would you *least* expect to see during prolonged space flight?**
   - **A.** Atrophy of the heart
   - **B.** Loss of bone mass
   - **C.** Nausea and vomiting
   - **D.** Increased circulating lymphocytes
   - **E.** Atrophy of skeletal muscles

Ans. **(D)**

Explanation:

Space motion sickness (nausea, vomiting and vertigo that occurs in astronauts), when they are just exposed to microgravity and often wears off after a few days of space flight.

Prolonged stay in space leads to:

1. Decrease in blood volume.
2. Steady loss of bone mineral with increased Ca^{+2} excretion.
3. Loss of red cell mass.
4. Alterations in plasma lymphocytes.

(Pg. 632)

8. **Which of the following takes longest to return to normal after 1 L of blood is removed from a normal individual?**
   - **A.** Plasma aldosterone concentration
   - **B.** Blood pressure
   - **C.** Renin secretion
   - **D.** Plasma volume
   - **E.** Number of red blood cells in peripheral blood

Ans. **(E)**

Explanation:

- After a moderate hemorrhage, circulating plasma volume is restored in 12-72 hours.
- Plasma albumin (protein) losses are replaced by hepatic synthesis over a period of 3-4 days.

- Erythropoietin appears in circulation and reticulocyte count increases reaching a peak in 10 days.
- Red cell mass is restored to normal in 4-8 weeks. *(Pg. 638)*

9. Which of the following is *least* likely to cause sustained hypertension?

A. Chronically increased secretion of the adrenal medulla
B. Chronically increased secretion of the zona fasciculata and zona reticularis of the adrenal cortex
C. Chronically increased secretion of the zona glomerulosa of the adrenal cortex
D. Chronically increased secretion of the posterior pituitary gland
E. Chronic treatment with oral contraceptives

Ans. (E)

Explanation:

- Post-pituitary releases oxytocin and vasopressin in circulation.
- Vasopressin also raises blood pressure when administered in large doses in normal animals, but infusion of doses that produce the same plasma vasopressin levels produced by hemorrhage causes only a small increase in blood pressure because compensatory decrease in cardiac output occurs. *(Also see Chapter 32, Pg. 639)*

10. Which of the following is *not* increased during isotonic exercise?

A. Respiratory rate
B. Stroke volume
C. Heart rate
D. Total peripheral resistance
E. Systolic blood pressure

Ans. (D)

Explanation:

Isometric muscle contraction	*Isotonic muscle contraction*
1. HR (Heart rate) increases	1. Prompt HR increases.
2. Systolic and diastolic BP rises sharply.	2. Stroke volume increases markedly.
3. Stroke volume changes relatively little and blood flow to contracting muscles is reduced as a result of compression of their blood vessels.	3. Net fall in total peripheral resistance due to vasodilation in exercising muscles, **so systolic blood pressure rises only moderately whereas diastolic pressure remains unchanged** or falls.

(Pg. 633)

11. Which of the following are *incorrectly* paired?

A. Loss of blood: hypertension
B. Negative G: blackout
C. Increased cardiac output: exercise
D. Renal artery constriction: increased blood pressure
E. Decreased total peripheral resistance: fainting

Ans. (B)

Explanation:

Positive G causes black out. Due to exposure to positive G, blood is thrown into the lower part of the body. At acceleration producing more than 5 g, however vision fails (black out) in about 5 sec and unconsciousness follows immediately thereafter.

(Pg. 632)

12. Which of the following would you expect to decrease in a normal individual who stands quietly in the same position for 1 hour?

A. Hematocrit
B. Diameter of the thigh

C. Plasma renin activity
D. Plasma vasopressin concentration
E. Central venous pressure

Ans. (E)

Explanation:

Mean arterial blood pressure in the feet of a normal adult =180-200 mm Hg
Venous pressure = 85-90 mm kg
If the individual does not move, 300-500 ml of blood pools in the venous capacitance vessels of the lower extremities, fluid begins of accumulate in interstitial spaces because of increased hydrostatic pressures in the capillaries and stroke volume is decreased.

(Pg. 630-631)

13. Which of the following is *least* likely to cause fainting?

A. Pressure on the carotid sinus
B. Autonomic insufficiency
C. Strong emotion
D. Acute myocardial infarction
E. Chronic congestive heart failure

Ans. (E)

Explanation:

Neurogenic shock can be:

1. **Vasovagal shock.**
2. **Postural syncope** due to prolonged standing.
3. **Micturition syncope** occurs in patients during fainting, in patients with orthostatic hypotension.
4. **Carotid sinus syncope**: Pressure on carotid sinus causes marked bradycardia and vasodilatation that fainting result.
5. **Deglutition syncope**: Vasodilatation and bradycardia may be precipitated by swallowing.
6. **Cough syncope**: Increased intrathoracic pressure causes block in venous return.

7. **Effort syncope** as a result of exertion, inability to meet cardiac output.
8. **Cardiac origin** due to sudden decrease in cardiac output or obstruction of blood flow to heart.

Fainting due to bradycardia, Heart block or sinus arrest is called **Neurocardiogenic syncope.** Fainting is present in 7% of patients with myocardial infarction. *(Pg. 640)*

14. Amount of NF-κB in cell nuclei after infusion of epinephrine is:

A. Greater than the amount of NF-κB in cell nuclei after infusion of cortisol
B. Same as the amount of NF-κB in cell nuclei after infusion of cortisol
C. Less than the amount of NF-κB in cell nuclei after infusion of cortisol

Ans. (A)

Explanation:

A transcription factor, nuclear factor κB, plays a key role in the inflammatory response, during local injury. Glucocorticoids inhibit activation of NF-κB by increasing the production of Iκ-Bα and this is probably the main basis of their anti-inflammatory action. *(Pg. 636)*

15. Total blood flow to brain during exercise.

A. Greater than the total blood flow to brain at rest
B. Same as the total blood flow to brain at rest
C. Less than the total blood flow to brain at rest

Ans. (B)

Explanation:

During exercise, blood flow to brain remains same = 750 ml/min.

	Quiet standing ml/min	*Isotonic exercise*
Cardiac output	25900	24,000
Blood flow to		
Heart	250	1000
Brain	750	750
Active skeletal muscle	650	20, 850
Inactive skeletal muscle	650	300
Skin	500	500
Kidney, liver, GIT, etc	3100	600

(Pg. 634)

Chapter 34 Pulmonary Function

1. On the summit of Mt. Everest, where the barometric pressure is about 250 mm Hg, the partial pressure of O_2 is about:

A. 0.1 mm Hg
B. 0.5 mm Hg
C. 5 mm Hg
D. 50 mm Hg
E. 100 mm Hg

Ans. (D)

Explanation:

The composition of dry air is:
20.98%: O_2
0.04%: CO_2
78.06% : N_2
0.92% : Inert gases (argon and helium)
Barometric pressure at sea level:
760 mm Hg (1 atmosphere)
The partial pressure of O_2 in dry air:
therefore 0.21 × 760= or 160 mm Hg at sea level
and 0.21 × 250 = 50 mm Hg at Mount Everest
(Pg. 647)

2. The approximate amount of gas left in the lungs after maximal forced expiration in a normal woman is:

A. Zero
B. 0.1 L
C. 1.1 L
D. 3.1 L
E. 4.2 L

Ans. (C)

Explanation:

Amount of air left in the lungs after a maximal forced expiration in a normal adult human is called as **Residual volume.**

In adult males: 1.2 L

In adult females: 1.1 L *(Pg. 652)*

3. The tidal volume in a normal man at rest is about:

A. 0.5 L
B. 1.2 L
C. 2.5 L
D. 4.9 L
E. 6.0 L

Ans. (A)

Explanation:

Tidal volume: Amount of air that moves into the lungs with each inspiration (or the amount of air that moves out with each expiration) during relaxed, quiet breathing. Tidal volume in men and women: 0.5 L.

4. What is the approximate dead space of a normal 70 kg man breathing through a tube that has a radius of 5 mm and a length of 100 cm?

A. 150 mL
B. 180 mL
C. 230 mL
D. 280 mL
E. 350 mL

Ans. (C)

Explanation:

1 kg = 2.2 lb.
70 kg = approximately 154 ml.
Normally the volume of dead space is approximately equal to the body weight in pounds, therefore, dead space in a 70 kg man = 154 ml.

- Adding a tube has a radius of 5 mm and length of 100 cm means we are adding a total volume of ($\pi r^2L = 3 \times 25 \times 1000 = 75000$ ml).
- 75000 ml of dead space where no exchange of gases will occur, so
  Total dead space volume = 154.0 ml + 75 ml
  = 229 ml.

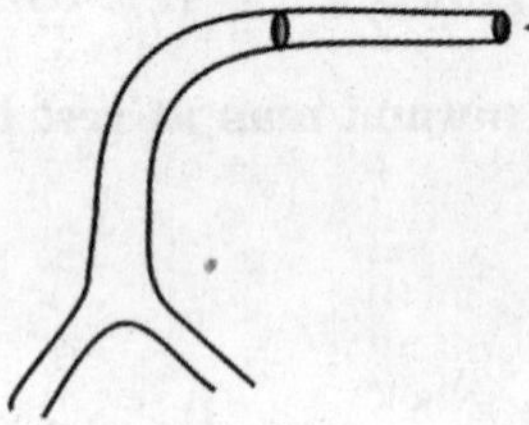

5. **Which of the following is responsible for the movement of O_2 from the alveoli into the blood in the pulmonary capillaries?**
   A. Active transport
   B. Filtration
   C. Secondary active transport
   D. Facilitated diffusion
   E. Passive diffusion

Ans. (E)

Explanation:

Gases diffuse from the alveoli to the blood in the pulmonary capillaries or vice-versa across the thin alveolo-capillary membrane made up of the pulmonary epithelium, capillary endothelium and their fused basement membranes. *(Pg. 660)*

Questions 6-8 refer to figure below:

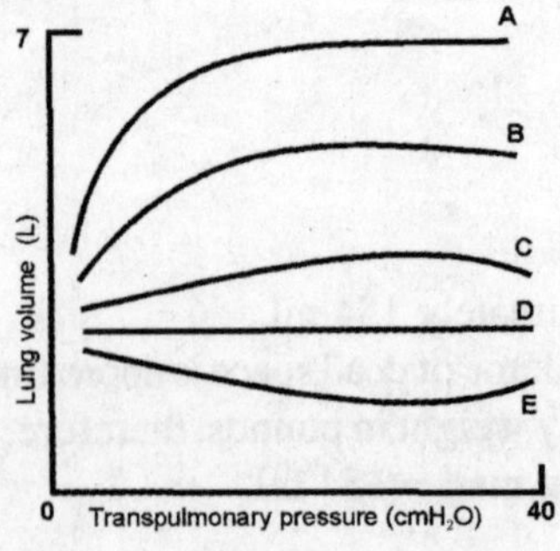

6. Which of the labeled curves would you expect to see in a normal individual?

Ans. (B)

7. Which of the labeled curves would you expect to see in a patient with severe pulmonary fibrosis?

Ans. (C)

8. Which of the labeled curves would you expect to see in a patient with advanced emphysema?

Ans. (A)

Explanation:

- Change in lung volume per unit change in airway pressure is the stretchability (compliance) of the lungs and chest wall.
- Compliance is studied by pressure-volume curve.
- Compliance is decreased (curve is shifted downward and to right) by **pulmonary congestion** and **interstitial pulmonary fibrosis.**
- Compliance is increased (curve is shifted upward and to left) in emphysema.

(Pg. 654-655)

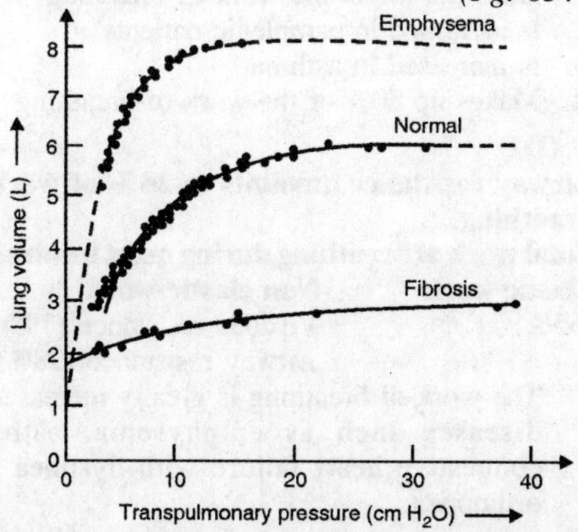

9. Which of the following causes relaxation of bronchial smooth muscle?

A. Leukotrienes
B. Vasoactive intestinal polypeptide (VIP)
C. Acetylcholine
D. Cool air
E. Sulfur dioxide

Ans. (B)

Explanation:

- Dilation is produced by sympathetic discharge.
- Constriction is produced by parasympathetic discharge.
- Stimulation of sensory receptors in airways by irritants and chemicals such as sulfur dioxide produce reflex bronchoconstriction that is mediated by cholinergic pathways.
- Cool air also causes bronchoconstriction, so does exercise.
- VIP (Vasoactive intestinal peptide) produces **bronchodilation.**
- Bronchoconstrictors { - Substance P, - Adenosine }

(Pg. 654)

10. Airway resistance:

A. Is increased if the lungs are removed and inflated with saline
B. Does not affect the work of breathing
C. Is increased in paraplegic patients
D. Is increased in asthma
E. Makes up 80% of the work of breathing

Ans. (D)

Airway resistance amounts to 28% of work of breathing.

Total work of breathing during quiet inspiration

Elastic work	**Non elastic work**
(65%)	Viscous resistance (7%)
	Airway resistance (28%)

- The work of breathing is greatly increased in diseases such as emphysema, asthma, congestive heart failure with dyspnea and orthopnea.

(Pg. 657)

In questions 11-13, one or more than one of the answers may be correct. Select:

A. If (1), (2) and (3) are correct
B. If (1) and (3) are correct
C. If (2) and (4) are correct
D. If only (4) is correct
E. If all are correct

11. Surfactant lining the alveoli:

1. Helps prevent alveolar collapse
2. Is decreased in hyaline membrane disease
3. Is decreased in the lungs of heavy smokers
4. Is a mixture of proteins and lipids

Ans. (E)

Explanation:

- Surfactant, a lipid surface-tension-lowering agent.
- It is a mixture of dipalmitoyl phosphatidylcholine (DPPC), other lipids and proteins.
- It helps prevent pulmonary edema.
- It is produced by type II alveolar epithelium cells.
- It is important at birth. The fetus makes respiratory movement in utero, but the lungs remain collapsed until birth. After birth, the infant makes several strong inspiratory movements and the lungs expand. Surfactant keeps them from collapsing again. Surfactant deficiency is an important cause of infant respiratory distress syndrome (IRDS or hyaline membrane disease), the serious pulmonary disease that develops in infants born before their surfactant system is functional.
- **Cigarette smoking** decreases lung surfactant.

12. Activation of which of the following receptors causes constriction of pulmonary arteries?

1. Adrenergic α_2 receptors
2. Muscarinic M_3 receptors
3. Histamine H_2 receptors
4. Endothelin ETA receptors

Ans. (D)

Explanation:

Receptors affecting smooth muscle in pulmonary arteries and veins

Receptor *Autonomic*	*Subtype*	*Response*	*Endothelium dependency*
1. Adrenergic	α_1	Contraction	No
	α_2	Relaxation	Yes
	β_2	Relaxation	Yes
2. Muscarinic	M_3	Relaxation	Yes
3. VIP	-	Relaxation	-
Humoral			
1. Adenosine	A_1	Contraction	No
	A_2	Relaxation	No
2. Histamine	H_1	Relaxation	Yes
	H_2	Relaxation	No
3. Endothelium	ET_A	Contraction	No
	ET_B	Relaxation	Yes

(Pg. 664)

13. Which of the following would be expected to cause a reduction in pulmonary ventilation?

1. Transection of both phrenic nerves
2. Transection of the spinal cord at the first thoracic level
3. A large dose of morphine
4. A broken rib

Ans. (E)

Explanation:

Either the diaphragm or the external intercostal muscles alone can maintain adequate ventilation at rest. Transection of the spinal cord above the 3rd cervical segment is fatal without artificial respiration, but transaetion below the 5th cervical segment is not, because it leaves the phrenic nerves that innervate the diaphragm intact (Root value of phrenic nerves (C_3, C_4, C_5). So patients with bilateral phrenic nerve palsy but intact innervation of their intercostal muscles, respiration is somewhat labored, but adequate to maintain life.

(Pg. 635)

14. FEV_1 in a normal individual is:

A. Greater than the FEV_1 in a patient with asthma
B. Same as the FEV_1 in a patient with asthma
C. Less than the FEV_1 in a patient with asthma

Ans. (A)

Explanation:

FEV_1

The fraction of the vital capacity expired during the first second of a forced expiration is reduced in asthma, in which airway resistance is increased because of bronchial constriction. *(Pg. 652)*

15. Angiotensin II concentration in blood in pulmonary veins is:

A. Greater than the angiotensin II concentration in blood in renal veins

B. Same as the angiotensin II concentration in blood in renal veins

C. Less than the angiotensin II concentration in blood in renal veins

Ans. (A)

Explanation:

Large amount of angiotensin converting enzyme (ACE) responsible for activation of angiotensin II is located on the surface of the endothelial cells of the pulmonary capillaries. Much of the conversion occurs when blood passes through lungs.

(Pg. 455, 665)

Chapter 35 Gas Transport Between the Lungs and the Tissues

1. Most of the CO_2 transported in the blood is:

A. Dissolved in plasma
B. In carbamino compounds formed from plasma proteins
C. In carbamino compounds formed from hemoglobin
D. Bound to Cl^-
E. In HCO_3^-

Ans. (E)

Explanation:

1. Transport of CO_2 in the dissolved state approximately 7%.
2. Transport of CO_2 in the form of bicarbonate ion approximately 70% (The reversible combination of CO_2 with H_2O in the RBC under the influence of carbonic anhydrase).
3. Transport of CO_2 in combination with hemoglobin and plasma proteins (carbamino hemoglobin) approximately 20%.

(Guyton, 11th Ed., Pg. 511)

2. Which of the following has the greatest effect on the ability of blood to transport oxygen?

A. Capacity of the blood to dissolve oxygen
B. Amount of hemoglobin in the blood
C. pH of plasma
D. CO_2
E. Temperature of the blood

Ans. (B)

Explanation:

Normally about 97% of the oxygen transported from the lungs to the tissues is carried in chemical combination with hemoglobin in RBC. The remaining 3% is transported in dissolved state in the water of the plasma and blood cells. The dynamics of reaction of hemoglobin with O_2 make it a particularly suitable O_2 carrier.

(Guyton, 11th Ed, Pg. 505)

3. Which of the following is not true of the system?

$$CO_2 + H_2O \rightleftarrows H_2CO_3 \rightleftarrows H^+ HCO_3^-$$

A. Reaction 1 is catalyzed by carbonic anhydrase
B. Because of reaction 2, the pH of blood declines during breath holding
C. Reaction 1 occurs in the kidneys
D. Reaction 1 occurs primarily in plasma
E. The reactions move to the left when there is excess H^+ in the tissues

Ans. (D)

Explanation:

The reversible combination of CO_2 with water in the RBC under the influence of carbonic anhydrase accounts for about 70% of the CO_2 transported from the tissues to the lungs.

In questions 4-7, select:

A. If the item is associated with (a) below
B. If the item is associated with (b) below
C. If the item is associated with both (a) and (b) below
D. If the item is associated with neither (a) nor (b)

(a) Involved in O_2 transport in blood
(b) Involved in CO_2 transport in blood

4. Carbamino compounds:

Ans. (B) See Ans. of question 1.

5. Myoglobin:

Ans. (D)

Explanation:

- Myoglobin is an iron-containing pigment found in skeletal muscle.
- It resembles hemoglobin but binds 1 rather than 4 molecules of O_2 per mole.

6. Hydrogen ions:

Ans. (C) See Ans. of question 1.

7. Plasma proteins:

Ans. (C) See Ans. of question 1.

8. Affinity of fetal hemoglobin (HbF) for O_2 is:

A. Greater than the affinity of adult hemoglobin (HbA) for O_2

B. Same as the affinity of adult hemoglobin (HbA) for O_2

C. Less than the affinity of adult hemoglobin (HbA) for O_2

Ans. (A)

Explanation:

The affinity of fetal hemoglobin (HbF) for O_2 which is greater than that for adult hemoglobin (Hb), facilitates the movement of O_2 from mother to fetus. The cause is poor binding of 2, 3BPG by γ polypeptide chains that replace β chains in fetal hemoglobin leading to greater affinity. *(Pg. 669)*

9. Number of osmotically active particles in red blood cells (RBC) in arterial blood is:

A. Greater than the number of osmotically active particles in RBC in venous blood

B. Same as the number of osmotically active particles in RBC in venous blood

C. Less than the number of osmotically active particles in RBC in venous blood

Ans. (C)

Explanation:

That for each CO_2 molecule added to the RBC, there is an increase of one osmotically active particle in the cell—either an HCO_3^- or a Cl^- in the RBC.

(Pg. 670)

Chapter 36 Regulation of Respiration

1. **The main respiratory control neurons:**
   - A. Send out regular bursts of impulses to expiratory muscles during quiet respiration
   - B. Are unaffected by stimulation of pain receptors
   - C. Are located in the pons
   - D. Send out regular bursts of impulses to inspiratory muscles during quiet respiration
   - E. Are unaffected by impulses from the cerebral cortex

Ans. **(D)**

Explanation:

Two separate neural mechanisms regulate respiration. One is responsible for voluntary control and the other for automatic control. The **voluntary control** is located in the cerebral cortex and sends impulses to the respiratory motor neurons via the corticospinal tracts. The **automatic system** is driven by a group of pacemaker cells in the medulla. Impulses from these cells activate motor neurons in the cervical and thoracic spinal cord that innervate inspiratory muscles. Those in the cervical cord activate the diaphragm via phrenic nerves and those in the thoracic spinal cord activate the external intercostal muscles.

(Pg. 671)

2. **Intravenous lactic acid increases ventilation. The receptors responsible for this effect are located in the:**
   - A. Medulla oblongata
   - B. Carotid bodies
   - C. Lung parenchyma
   - D. Aortic baroreceptors
   - E. Trachea and large bronchi

Ans. (B)

Explanation:

The receptors in the carotid and aortic bodies are stimulated by a rise in the **PCO_2** or **H^+ conc.** of **arterial blood** or a decline in **its PO_2**. *(Pg. 672)*

3. **Spontaneous respiration ceases after:**
   A. Transection of the brainstem above the pons
   B. Transection of the brainstem at the caudal end of the medulla
   C. Bilateral vagotomy
   D. Bilateral vagotomy combined with transection of the brainstem at the superior border of the pons
   E. Transection of the spinal cord at the level of the first thoracic segment

Ans. (B)

Explanation:

Rhythmic respiration is initiated by a small group of synaptically coupled pacemaker cells in the **pre-Botzinger complex (pre-BOTC)** on either side of the medulla between the nucleus ambiguous (NA) and the lateral reticular nucleus (LRN). These neurons discharge rhythmically and produce rhythmic discharges in the phrenic motor neurons (Supply diaphragm).

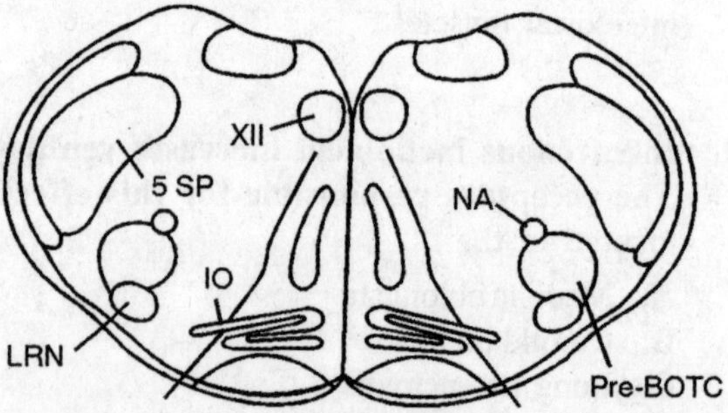

- Stretching of lungs during inspiration initiates impulses in the afferent pulmonary vagal fibers. These impulses inhibit inspiratory discharge. This is why the depth of inspiration is increased after **vagotomy** and **apneusis** develops if vagi are cut after damage to the pneumotaxic center.

4. The following physiologic events that occur in vivo are listed in random order:

1. Decreased cerebrospinal fluid pH
2. Increased arterial fluid PCO_2
3. Increased cerebrospinal fluid PCO_2
4. Stimulation of medullary chemoreceptors
5. Increased alveolar PCO_2

What is the usual sequence in which they occur when they affect respiration?

A. 1, 2, 3, 4, 5
B. 4, 1, 3, 2, 5
C. 3, 4, 5, 1, 2
D. 5, 2, 3, 1, 4
E. 5, 3, 2, 4, 1

Ans. (D)

Explanation:

The chemoreceptors that mediate the hyperventilation produced by increases in **arterial PCO_2** after carotid and aortic bodies are denervated are located in medulla oblongata and consequently are called **medullarly chemoreceptors.**

- Located on ventral surface of medulla.
- Monitor H^+ concentration of **CSF**, including the brain **interstitial fluid.**
- CO_2 readily penetrates membranes, including blood-brain barrier, whereas H^+ and HCO_3^- penetrate slowly.

Therefore, effects of CO_2 on respiration are mainly due to its movement into CSF and brain interstitial fluid → increases H^+ concentration → stimulates receptors sensitive to H^+.

(Pg. 675)

5. **The following events that occur in the carotid bodies when they are exposed to hypoxia are listed in random order:**
   1. Depolarization of type I glomus cells
   2. Excitation of afferent nerve endings
   3. Reduced conductance of hypoxia-sensitive K^+ channels in type I glomus cells
   4. Ca^{+2} entry into type I glomus cells
   5. Decreased K^+ efflux

   What is the usual sequence in which they occur on exposure to hypoxia?

   A. 1, 3, 4, 5, 2
   B. 1, 4, 2, 5, 3
   C. 3, 4, 5, 1, 2
   D. 3, 1, 4, 5, 2
   E. 3, 5, 1, 4, 2

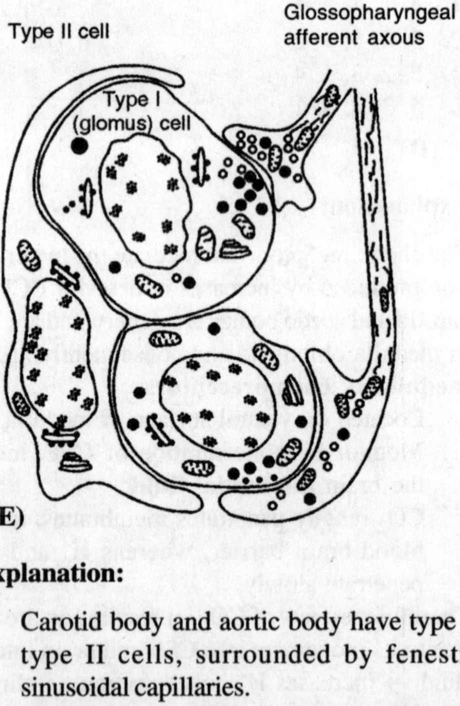

Ans. (E)

Explanation:

- Carotid body and aortic body have type I and type II cells, surrounded by fenestrated sinusoidal capillaries.
- Glomus/type I cells have catecholamines which γ are released upon exposure to hypoxia and cyanide.

- Type I cells have O_2 sensitive K^+ channels, whose conductance is reduced in proportion to degree of hypoxia to which they are exposed.
- This decrease K^+ efflux leading to depolarization which causes Ca^{+2} influx via L-type Ca^{+2} channels. This Ca^{+2} influx triggers action potentials which cause transmitter release leading to excitation of afferent nerve endings.

(Pg. 674)

Important Feature

- Smooth muscle of pulmonary arteries contains similar O_2 sensitive K^+ channels which mediate **vasoconstriction** caused by hypoxia.
- This is in **contrast** to **systemic arteries** which contain ATP dependent K^+ channels that permit more K^+ efflux with hypoxia and so **vasodilation** instead of constriction.

6. Stimulation of the central (proximal) end of a cut vagus nerve would be expected to:

A. Increase heart rate
B. Stimulate inspiration
C. Inhibit coughing
D. Raise blood pressure
E. Cause apnea

Ans. (E)

Explanation:

When vagus is cut, there are prolonged inspiratory spasms that resemble breath holding (apneusis) because stretching of lungs during inspiration, initiates impulses in afferent pulmonary vagal fibers, which inhibit inspiratory discharge. That is why the depth of inspiration is increased after vagotomy and apneusis develops if the vagi are cut after damage to the pneumotaxic center.

(Pg. 671-672)

7. Injection of a drug that stimulates the carotid bodies would be expected to cause:

A. A decrease in the pH of arterial blood
B. A decrease in PCO_2 of arterial blood
C. An increase in the HCO_3^- concentration of arterial blood
D. An increase in urinary Na^+ excretion
E. An increase in plasma Cl^-

Ans. (B)

Explanation:

The chemical regulatory mechanisms (carotid and aortic bodies) adjust ventilation in such a way that the alveolar PCO_2 is normally held constant, the effects of H^+ in the blood are combated and PO_2 is raised when it falls to a potentially dangerous levels. *(Pg. 672)*

8. Variations in which of the following components of blood or cerebrospinal fluid to *not* affect respiration?

A. Arterial HCO_3^- concentration
B. Arterial H^+ concentration
C. Arterial Na^+ concentration
D. Cerebrospinal fluid CO_2 concentration
E. Cerebrospinal fluid H^+ concentration

Ans. (C)

Explanation:

The effects of increased PCO_2 (arterial) on respiration is mainly due to movement into CSF and brain intestinal fluid, where it increases H^+ concentration and stimulates receptor sensitive to H^+. *(Pg. 675)*

9. Intractable hiccups sometimes respond to:

A. Increasing arterial PO_2
B. Injection of acetylcholine

C. Injection of dopamine antagonists
D. Increasing arterial pH
E. Hyperventilation

Ans. (C)

Explanation:

Most attacks of hiccups are usually of short duration and they often respond to breathholding or other measures that increase arterial PCO_2. Intractable hiccups which can be debilitating, sometimes respond to dopamine antagonists and perhaps to some centrally acting analgesic compounds.

(Pg. 680)

10. Proportion of the alteration in ventilation produced by changes in arterial PCO_2 that is due to medullary chemoreceptors:

A. Greater than the proportion of the alteration in ventilation produced by changes in arterial PCO_2 that is due to peripheral chemoreceptors
B. Same as the proportion of the alteration in ventilation produced by changes in arterial PCO_2 that is due to peripheral chemoreceptors
C. Less than the proportion of the alteration in ventilation produced by changes in arterial PCO_2 that is due to peripheral chemoreceptors

Ans. (A)

Explanation:

The direct effect of CO_2 concentration/H^+ ion concentration on respiratory center itself is much more powerful than their effects mediated via chemoreceptors (7 times more powerful). But the stimulation by peripheral chemoreceptors (carotid body and aortic bodies) occurs 5 times more rapidly as central stimulation so that peripheral chemoreceptors might be especially important in increasing the rapidity of response to CO_2 at the onset of exercise.

(Guyton, 11th Ed, Pg. 578)

11. Blood flow per gram of tissue to carotid bodies is:

A. Greater than the blood flow per gram of tissue to brain

B. Same as the blood flow per gram of tissue to brain

C. Less than the blood flow per gram of tissue to brain

Ans. (A)

Explanation:

Blood flow in each 2 mg carotid body is about 0.04 ml/min or 2000 ml/100 g of tissue/min

So

Carotid body	Blood flow
	2000 ml/100 g of tissue/min
Brain	54 ml/100 g/min
Kidneys	420 ml/100 g/min

Chapter 37 Respiratory Adjustments in Health and Disease

In questions 1-16, select the single best answer. Questions 1-5 refer to the following Table.

PO_2 (mm Hg)

	Superior vena cava	*Right ventricle*	*Alveolar gas*	*Left ventricle*
A	45	40	104	94
B	40	35	105	94
C	40	35	60	55
D	40	35	104	55
E	45	80	104	94

1. Which set of data would you expect to find in a normal person?

Ans. (B)

- The PO_2 of **alveolar** air is normally : 100 mm Hg
- The PO_2 of **blood** entering pulmonary capillaries (right side of heart) : 40 mm Hg

The PO_2 of blood entering left side : 97 mm Hg
of heart but falls to : 95 mm Hg **(due to physiologic shunt)**

(Pg. 661)

2. Which set of data would you expect to find in a person at rest breathing air at an altitude of 3000 m (10,000 feet; barometric pressure= 520 mm Hg)?

Ans. (C)

Explanation:

At 3000 m (approximately 10,000 feet) above sea level, the alveolar PO_2 is **60 mm Hg** and there is enough hypoxic stimulation of the chemoreceptor to definitely increase ventilation. *(Pg. 684)*

3. Which set of data would you expect to find in a patient with a large left-to-right shunt?

Ans. (E)

Explanation:

Better oxygenation on right side of the heart.

4. Which set of data would you expect to find in a patient with a collapsed lung?

Ans. (D)

Explanation:

In case of collapsed lung, same blood is diverted from the collapsed area to better ventilated portions of the lung, and this reduces the magnitude of the decline in arterial PO_2.

5. Which set of data would you expect to find in a normal subject at rest breathing 100% O_2 in an unpressurized airplane cabin at 10,000 m (32, 800 feet; barometric pressure= 180 mm Hg)?

Ans. (A) *(Guyton, Table 43.1, 11th Ed, Pg. 538)*

Explanation:

Breathing pure O_2

Altitude (feet)	PCO_2 in alveoli (mmHg)	PO_2 in alveoli (mmHg)	Arterial O_2 saturation (100%)
0	40	673	100
10,000	40	436	100
20,000	40	262	100
30,000	40	139	99
40,000	36	58	84
50,000	24	16	15

Questions 6 and 7 refer the following Table.

Arterial blood valves

	PCO_2 (mmHg)	Ph	HCO_3^- (meq/l)
A	60	7.25	29
B	25	7.30	12
C	42	7.55	35
D	25	7.50	20
E	60	7.05	15

6. Which set of data would you expect to find in a man who is breathing through a tube that greatly increases his dead space?

Ans. (A)

Explanation:

Increase in dead space, increases PCO_2 levels decreasing pH of body fluids.
(Normal pH: 7.35 - 7.45)
(Normal HCO_3: 28meq/l ECF)

7. Which set of data would you expect to find in a woman who is flying at an altitude of 4500 m (14750 ft) breathing air in the open cockpit of an airplane?

Ans. (D)

Explanation:

The immediate increase in pulmonary renulation in rising to a high altitude blows off large quantities of CO_2, reducing PCO_2 and increasing the pH of body fluids.

(Guyton, 11th Ed., Pg. 539)

8. In which of the following conditions is CO_2 retention most likely to occur?

A. Climbing a high mountain
B. Metabolic acidosis
C. Carbon monoxide poisoning
D. Ventilatory failure
E. Hysterical hyperventilation

Ans. (D) *(Pg. 684)*

9. Pulmonary fibrosis would be expected to produce:

A. Histotoxic hypoxia
B. Stagnant hypoxia
C. Decreased vital capacity
D. Cyanosis
E. Emphysema

Ans. (D)

Explanation:

Cyanosis, the bluish discoloration of the tissues appears when the amount of **reduced** hemoglobin concentration of blood in capillaries is > 5g/dl.

- Its **occurrence** depends on:
  - Total amount of hemoglobin in blood.
  - Degree of hemoglobin unstauration.
  - State of the capillary circulation.
- It **does not** occur in:
  - Anaemic hypoxia.
  - CO poisoning.
  - Histotoxic hypoxia.

10. Which of the following deleterious effects would probably *not* be produced by chronic cigarette smoking?

A. Patches of atelectasis
B. Myocardial ischemia
C. Loss of elastic tissue in the lung
D. Increased anatomic dead space
E. Increased carbonmonoxyhemoglobin in blood

Ans. (E)

Explanation:

Cigarette smoking produces emphysema. *(Pg. 689)*

Causes:

- Smoke causes an increase in the number of pulmonary alveolar macrophages, these macrophages release a chemical, substance that attracts leukocytes to the lungs. Leukocytes in turn release proteases including **elastase**, which attacks elastic tissue in lungs.

- At same time α1-antitrypsin that normally causes inactivation of elastase and other proteases is also inhibited.
- α_1-antitrypsin is inactivated by oxygen radicals and these are released by leukocytes.
- The final result is a protease-antiprotease imbalance→ with increased destruction of lung tissue. *(Pg. 689)*

11. O_2 delivery to the tissues would be reduced to the greater extent in:

A. A normal subject breathing 100% O_2 on top of Mt. Everest
B. A normal subject running a marathon at sea level
C. A patient with carbon monoxide poisoning
D. A patient who has ingested cyanide
E. A patient with moderately severe metabolic acidosis.

Ans. (C) *(Pg. 690)*

Explanation:

CO is toxic because it vest will hemoglobin to form carbonmonoxyhemoglobin (COHb or carboxyhemoglobin) and COHb cannot take up O_2.

12. Which of the following is not a manifestation of oxygen toxicity?

A. Irritation of the respiratory tract
B. Difficulty in seeing because of retrolental fibroplasia
C. Convulsions
D. Lung cysts in infants
E. Rapture of the deep

Ans. (E) *(Pg. 691)*

Explanation:

When 80-100% O_2 is administered to human for period of 8 hours or more, the respiratory passages become irritated, causing:

- Substernal distress
- Nasal congesting
- Sore throat and coughing.

Some infants treated with O_2 for respiratory disease syndrome develop a chronic condition characterized by lung cysts and densities **(Bronchopulmonary, dysphasia)**.

- Another complication is **Retinopathy of prematurely (Retrolental fibroplasias)** the formation of opaque vascular tissue in the eyes, which can lead to serious usual defects.

13. Which of the following drugs would be most useful in treating high-altitudę illness?

A. Erythropoietin
B. Spironolactone
C. Erythromycin
D. Amiloride
E. Acetazolamide

Ans. (E)

Explanation:

Acetazolamide inhibits carbonic anhydrase producing:

1. Increased HCO_3^- excretion in the urine.
2. Stimulating respiration.
3. Increasing $PaCO_2$; and
4. Reducing formation of CSF. *(Pg. 686)*

In questions 14-18, match the item in each question with the lettered disease most closely associated with it. Each lettered disease may be selected once, more than once, or not at all.

A. Asthma
B. Pulmonary hypertension
C. Emphysema
D. Cystic fibrosis
E. Acute respiratory distress syndrome

14. Shock:

Ans. (E)

15. Cigarette smoking:

Ans. (C)

Explanation:

Causes:

- Smoke causes an increase in the number of pulmonary alveolar macrophages, these macrophages release a chemical, substance that attracts leukocytes to the lungs. Leukocytes in turn release proteases including **elastase**, which attacks elastic tissue in lungs.
- At same time α_1-antitrypsin that normally causes inactivation of elastase and other proteases is also inhibited.
- α_1-antitrypsin is inactivated by oxygen radicals and these are released by leukocytes.
- The final result is a protease-antiproteases imbalance → with increased destruction of lung tissue.

16. Abnormal folding of a key protein:

Ans. (D)

Explanation:

Cystic fibrosis: Gene that is abnormal is located on chromosome 7 and encodes cystic fibrosis transmembrane conductance regulator (CFTR), regulated Cl^- channel.

- The most common mutation causing cystic fibrosis is loss of phenylalanine residue of protein (▲F 508), which hinders proper folding of the molecule leading to its more rapid destruction. *(Pg. 689)*

17. Denuding of airway epithelium:

Ans. (A)

Explanation:

Three abnormalities are present in asthma:

1. Airway obstruction that is at least partially reversible.
2. Airway inflammation.
3. Airway hyper responsiveness to a variety of stimuli.

   Proteins released from eosinophils in the inflammatory reaction may damage the airway epithelium and contribute to hyper responsiveness. *(Pg. 689)*

18. Corpulmonale:

Ans. (B)

Explanation:

Enlargement of right side of heart (corpulmonale) due to pulmonary hypertension (usually seen in pulmonary disorders e.g. emphysema). *(Pg. 689)*

Chapter 38 Renal Function and Micturition

In questions 1-17, select the single best answer. In questions 1-5, which refer to Table below, match the disease or condition in each question with the lettered pattern of laboratory findings in the Table that is most closely associated with it. Each lettered pattern may be selected once, more than once, or not at all.

	24-hour urine Volume (L)	*Ketones*	*Glucose*	*Protein*
A	1.4	+	0	0
B	6.2	2+	4+	0
C	1.6	0	0	4+
D	6.4	0	0	0
E	0.4	0	0	0

1. Diabetes insipidus (DI):

Ans. (D)

Explanation:

Causes of DI:

The condition is caused by vasopressin deficiency or failure to respond to the hormone, the collecting duct epithelium is relatively:

- **Impermeable to water**. The fluid therefore remains hypotonic and large amounts flow into the renal pelvis.
- **Urine osmolality** may be as low as 30 mosm/kg of H_2O.
- As much as 13% of filtered water may be excreted and urine flow may reach 15 ml/min or more.

2. Nephrosis:

Ans. (C)

Explanation:

Nephrosis is associated with loss of protein in urine.

3. Fasting:

Ans. (A)

Explanation:

Normal blood ketone levels in humans is approximately 1 mg/dl and less than 1mg is excreted in 24 hours because ketones are normally metabolized as rapidly as they are formed.

- The conditions which lead to **deficient** intercellular glucose **supplies**, leads to accumulation of ketone bodies in blood stream (ketoacidosis).

E.g.

- Starvation.
- Diabetes mellitus.
- High fat, low carbohydrate diet.

4. Dehydration:

Ans. (E)

Explanation:

Dehydration:
Normal urine volume: approx. 1L/day.
So in dehydration: value falls.

5. Diabetes mellitus:

Ans. (B)

Explanation:

Diabetes mellitus:
Presence of large amount of unreabsorbed solutes in the renal tubules causes an increase in urine volume called **osmotic diuresis**. So in diabetes mellitus, glucose that remains in tubules when the filtered load exceeds the TmG causes **polyuria**.

- Due to deficient glucose supplies, ketone bodies accumulate leading to **ketoacidosis.** *(Pg. 719)*

6. In the presence of vasopressin, the greatest fraction of filtered water is absorbed in the:

A. Proximal tubule
B. Loop of Henle
C. Distal tubule
D. Cortical collecting duct
E. Medullary collecting duct

Ans. (A)

Explanation:

- 60-70% of filtered solute; and
- 60-70% of filtered water is reabsorbed in proximal tubule. *(Pg. 714)*

7. In the absence of vasopressin, the greatest fraction of filtered water is absorbed in the:

A. Proximal tubule
B. Loop of Henle
C. Distal tubule
D. Cortical collecting duct
E. Medullary collecting duct

Ans. (A)

8. If the clearance of a substance which is freely filtered is less than that of inulin:

A. There is net reabsorption of the substance in the tubules
B. There is net secretion of the substance in the tubules
C. The substance is neither secreted nor reabsorbed in the tubules
D. The substance becomes bound to protein in the tubules
E. The substance is secreted in the proximal tubule to a greater degree than in the distal tubule

Ans. (A)

9. Glucose reabsorption occurs in the:

A. Proximal tubule
B. Loop of Henle
C. Distal tubule
D. Cortical collecting duct
E. Medullary collecting duct

Ans. (A)

Explanation:

Glucose, amino acids and bicarbonate are reabsorbed along with Na^+ in the early portion of the proximal tubules. Essentially all of the glucose is reabsorbed and no more than a few mg appear in the urine per 24 hours. *(Pg. 709)*

10. On which of the following does aldosterone exert its greatest tubule?

A. Glomerulus
B. Proximal tubule
C. Thin portion of the loop of Henle
D. Thick portion of the loop of Henle
E. Cortical collecting duct

Ans (E)

Explanation:

Hormone	*Site of action*	*Effects*
Aldosterone	Principal cells of the cortical collecting tubule	Increased NaCl and H_2O reabsorption while increased K^+ secretion

Mode of action: Increase number of ENAC in collecting tubule (epithelial Na^+ channels)

11. What is the clearance of a substance when its concentration in the plasma is 10 mg/dL, its concentration in the urine is 100 mg/dL, and urine flow is 2 mL/min?

A. 2 mL/min
B. 10 mL/min

C. 20 mL/min
D. 200 mL/min
E. Clearance cannot be determined from the information given.

Ans. (C)

Explanation:

$$\text{Clearance} = \frac{U\,\text{Conc in (mg/dl)} \times V\,\text{(urine flow rate) ml/min}}{P\,\text{Plasma conc (mg/dl)}}$$

$$= \frac{100 \times 2}{10}$$

$$= 20 \text{ ml/min}$$

(Pg. 706)

12. As urine flow increases during osmotic diuresis:

A. The osmolality of urine falls below that of plasma
B. The osmolality of urine increases because of the increased amounts of non-reabsorbable solute in the urine
C. The osmolality of urine approaches that of plasma because plasma leaks into the tubules
D. The osmolality of urine approaches that of plasma because an increasingly large fraction of the excreted urine is isotonic proximal tubular fluid
E. The action of vasopressin on the renal tubules is inhibited

Ans. (D)

Explanation:

Solutes that are not reabsorbed, in the proximal tubules exert an appreciable osmotic effect as the volume of tubular fluid decreases and their concentration rises. Therefore they "hold water in the tubules." In addition the concentration gradient against which Na^+ can be pumped out of proximal tubules is limited. So Na^+ remains in the tubule and water stays along with it. The result is that the loop of Henle is presented with greatly increased volume of isotonic fluid. In the loop, reabsorption of water and Na^+ is decreased, because the medullary hypertonicity is decreased.

- The decrease in medullary hypertonicity is due to decreased reabsorption of Na^+, K^+ and Cl^- in the ascending limb of loop of Henle.
- More fluid passes through distal tubule and because of the decrease in osmotic gradient along the medullarly pyramids, less water is reabsorbed in the collecting ducts. The result is a marked increase in urine volume and excretion of Na^+ and other electrolytes.

(Pg. 719)

For Questions 13-15 refer to the data in the following Table which were obtained in a normal woman.

	Control period	*Experimental period*
Arterial Plasma		
Inulin (mg/mL)	0.004	0.004
Glucose (mg/dL)	100 (1 mg/ML)	300 (3 mg/mL)
Urea (mmol/mL)	5	5
Urine		
Inulin (mg/mL)	0.4	0.2
Glucose (mg/mL)	0	5
Urea (mmol/mL)	300	160
Urine flow (mL/min)	1	2

13. The glomerular filtration rate in the experimental period is:

A. Four times that in the control period
B. Twice that in the control period
C. The same as in the control period
D. One half that in the control period
E. One quarter that in the control period

Ans. (C)

U inulin conc in urine (mg/ml) ×
V (urine flow ml/min)

GFR = P plasma inulin conc(mg/ml)

Inulin clearance is used to measure GFR.

$$GFR = \frac{U \times V}{P} =$$

Therefore Control period $= \frac{0.4 \times 1}{0.004} = 100$ ml/min

In Experimental period

$$GFR = \frac{U \times V}{P} = \frac{0.2 \times 2}{0.004}$$

= 100 ml/min

14. The clearance of urea in the experimental period is:

A. Increased, probably because the urine flow is increased

B. Increased, probably because the urine glucose concentration is increased

C. The same as in the control period

D. Decreased, probably because the urine flow is increased

E. Decreased, probably because the amount of urea filtered is decreased

Ans. (A)

Explanation:

$$\text{Urea clearance} = \frac{\text{U urine conc. of urea (m mol/ml)} \times \text{V urine flow rate (ml/min)}}{\text{P plasma conc. of urea (m mol/ml)}}$$

Urea clearance (control period) $= \frac{300 \times 1}{5}$

= 66 ml/min

Urea clearance (experimental period) $= \frac{160 \times 2}{5}$

= 66 ml/min

So urine flow rate is increased, leading to more urea clearance in experimental period.

15. The Tm for glucose in this woman:

A. Is 100 mg/min
B. Is 130 mg/min
C. Is 200 mg/min
D. Is 290 mg/min
E. Cannot be calculated from the data given

Ans. **(D)**

Explanation:

Concentration of glucose in tubular fluid = 300 mg/dl

Concentration of glucose excreted = 5 mg/ml
Volume of urine excreted = 2 ml/min

Therefore total amount of glucose excreted per min=concentration of glucose excreted × volume of urine excreted = 5 × 2
=10 mg/min

Therefore total amount of glucose absorbed (TmG)= concentration of glucose in tubule-total glucose excreted

= 300–10
= 290 mg/min

16. To produce a concentrated urine, vasopressin:

A. Induces the movement of aquaporin from the cytoplasm to the cell membrane of proximal tubule cells
B. Increases the movement of aquaporin-2 from the cytoplasm to the cell membrane of collecting duct cells
C. Has no effect on molecular motors in proximal tubule cells
D. Has no effect no molecular motors in collecting duct cells
E. Increases Na^+ reabsorption in the thick ascending limb of Henle

Ans. **(B)**

Explanation:

The key to the action of vasopressin on the **collecting ducts** is **aquaporin-2**. This is stored in vesicles in the cytoplasm of **principal cells.** Vasopressin causes rapid insertion of these vesicles into the apical membrane of cells. *(Pg. 716)*

17. A gain-of-function mutation in the gene for which of the following proteins is associated with increased Na^+ retention and hypertension with a normal or low plasma aldosterone level (Liddle's syndrome)?

A. Aldosterone synthase
B. An inward rectifier K^+ channel
C. 11 β-Hydroxylase
D. V_2 receptor
E. Epithelial Na^+ channel

Ans. (E)

Explanation:

Liddle's syndrome: Mutations in the genes that code for ENAC (Epithelial Na^+ channels) cause them to become constitutively active in kidney. This leads to Na^+ retention and hypertension. *(Pg. 123)*

18. Which of the following causes the greatest increase in the amount of K^+ excreted in the urine?

A. Mannitol
B. Calcium chloride
C. Aldactone
D. Furosemide
E. Ethanol

Ans. (D)

Explanation:

Loop diuretics (Furosemide) inhibit $Na^+ - K^+ - 2\ Cl^-$ cotransporter in the thick segment of loop of Henle.

Therefore

- Cause marked natriuresis and kaliuresis (increased excretion of K^+).
- So prolonged use of them, leads to K^+ depletion and hypokalemia unless not supplemented by K^+ intake.
- **Mannitol** acts as osmotic diuretic which inhibits water and solute reabsorption.
- **Ethanol** inhibits vasopressin secretion.

(Pg. 725)

Questions 19-23 refer to Figure below. Select the letter or letters identifying the appropriate part of the nephron. Each lettered item may be selected once, more than once, or not at all. Note that in some instances, the correct answer may be more than one letter.

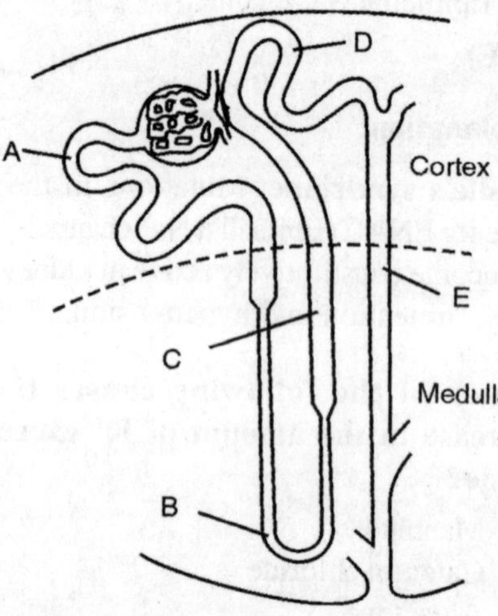

Juxtamedullary nephron

19. Site(s) at which furosemide acts:

Ans. (C)

Explanation:

Loop of Henle act as counter current multipliers, producing a gradient of hyperosmolarity in the medullary interstitium (MI).

20. Site(s) at which thiazides act:

Ans. (D)

Explanation:

Loop diuretics (Furosemide) act on thick ascending loop of Henle.

21. Site(s) at which tubular fluid osmolality exceeds that of plasma by the greatest amount:

Ans. (B)

Explanation:

Thiazide diuretics : act on early distal tubules.

22. Site(s) at which Na^+ is actively reabsorbed:

Ans. (A), (C), (D), (E)

Explanation:

Na^+ is actively reabsorbed in **proximal tubule, ascending limb of loop of Henle**, distal tubule and collecting ducts.
In **thick ascending limb**: Na^+ is cotransported from cells into interstitium by $Na^+ - K^+$ ATPase in basolateral membranes of cells.

See Table on the next page

23. Site(s) at which K^+ is secreted:

Ans. (D) and (E).

Aldosterone acts on collecting tubule (P cells) and duct where it increases Na^+ reabsorption while at the same time increasing potassium secretion by stimulating $Na^+ - K^+$ ATPase pump on the basolateral side of the cortical collecting tubule membrane.

(Guyton, 11th Ed., Pg. 342)

Summary of tubule characteristics—Urine concentration

	Active NaCl transport	*Permeability*		
		H_2O	*NaCl*	*Urea*
1. Proximal tubule	++	++	+	+
2. Thin descending limb	0	++	+	+
3. Thin ascending limb	0	0	+	+
4. Thick ascending limb	++	0	0	0
5. Distal tubule	+	+ADH	0	0
6. Cortical collecting tubule	+	+ADH	0	0
7. Inner medullary collecting duct	+	+ADH	0	++ADH

0 : minimal level of active transport/permeability.
+ : moderate level of active transport/permeability.
++ : high level of active transport/permeability.
+ADH : permeability to water/urea is increased by ADH.

(Guyton, 11th Ed., Pg. 351)

Chapter 39 Regulation of Extracellular Fluid Composition and Volume

Questions 1-4 refer to the numbered points on the nomogram in the following figure. Match the numbered point in each question with the lettered condition that is most closely associated with it. Each lettered condition may be selected once, more than once, or not at all.

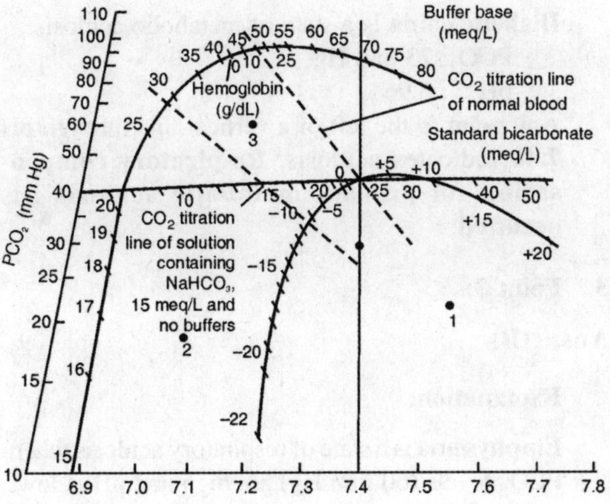

Siggard-Andersen curve nomogram

A. Values seen in a mountain climber after several weeks at high altitude
B. Values seen in long-standing severe emphysema
C. Values seen in diabetic coma
D. Values seen after 5 minutes of hyperventilation
E. Values seen after prolonged vomiting

1. Point 1:

Ans. (D)

Explanation:

- Any point below the horizontal line through a PCO_2 of 40 mmHg define effective degree of **hyperventilation.**
- Any point to the right of a vertical line through pH 7.40 indicates **alkalosis**. So state of Respiratory alkalosis. *(Pg. 736)*

2. **Point 2:**

Ans. (C)

Explanation:

Diabetic coma is a state of metabolic acidosis.

PCO_2: 23 mm Hg
pH : 6.96

Any point to the left of a vertical line through pH **7.40** indicates acidosis. **Respiratory compensation** for primary **metabolic** acidosis has occurred.

3. **Point 3:**

Ans. (B)

Explanation:

Emphysema is a state of respiratory acidosis where PCO_2 levels (60 mm Hg) are high and pH is low.

4. **Point 4:**

Ans. (A)

Explanation:

High altitude after several weeks

- pH : 7.48
- PCO_2: 26 mmHg.

After several weeks at high altitude, renal compensation for primary metabolic alkalosis will be made.

5. **Dehydration increases the plasma concentration of all the following hormones *except*:**
   - **A.** Vasopressin
   - **B.** Angiotensin II
   - **C.** Aldosterone
   - **D.** Norepinephrine
   - **E.** Atrial natriuretic peptide

Ans. (E)

Explanation:

Atrial natriuretic peptide acts on the kidneys to increase Na^+ excretion. *(Pg. 460)*

- **Vasopressin:** Acts on collecting tubules and helps in water reabsorption. *(Pg. 716)*
- **Angiotensin II:** Produces potent arteriolar constriction and a rise in systolic and diastolic blood pressure.
- Also acts directly on adrenal cortex to increase secretion of aldosterone. *(Pg. 458)*
- Aldosetrone increases amount of reabsorption of Na^+ ions and excretion of K^+ ions and H^+ producing K^+ diuresis and increase in urine acidity.
- NE (Norepinephrine) produces vasoconstriction in most if not all organs via α_1 receptors.

6. **Which of the following is the principal buffer in interstitial fluid?**
   - **A.** Hemoglobin
   - **B.** Other proteins
   - **C.** Carbonic acid
   - **D.** H_2PO_4
   - **E.** Compounds containing histidine

Ans. (C)

Explanation:

Principal buffers in body fluids:

Blood $H_2CO_3 \rightleftharpoons H^+ + HCO_3^-$

$HProt \rightleftharpoons H^+ + prot^-$

$HHb \rightleftharpoons H^+ + Hb^-$

Interstitial fluid $H_2CO_3 \rightleftharpoons H^+ + HCO_3^-$

Intercellular fluid $HProt \rightleftharpoons H^+ + Prot^-$

$H_2PO_4 \rightleftharpoons H^+ + HPO_4^{-2}$

(Pg. 733)

7. **Increasing alveolar ventilation increases the blood pH because:**
   A. It activates neural mechanisms that remove acid from the blood
   B. It makes hemoglobin a stronger acid
   C. It increases the PO_2 of the blood
   D. It decreases the PCO_2 in the alveoli
   E. The increased muscle work of increased breathing generates more CO_2

Ans. (D)

8. **In uncompensated metabolic alkalosis:**
   A. The plasma pH, the plasma HCO_3^- concentration, and the arterial PCO_2 are all low
   B. The plasma pH is high and the plasma HCO_3^- concentration and arterial PCO_2 are low
   C. The plasma pH and the plasma HCO_3^- concentration are low and the arterial PCO_2 is normal
   D. The plasma pH and the plasma HCO_3^- concentration are high and the arterial PCO_2 is normal
   E. The plasma pH is low, the plasma HCO_3^- concentration is high, and the arterial PCO_2 is normal

Ans. (D)

Explanation:

The plasma pH and the plasma HCO_3^- concentration are high and the arterial PCO_2 is normal. Rise or increase in plasma H^+ stimulates respiration, so that PCO_2, instead of rising or remaining constant is reduced. This respiratory compensation raises the pH even further. The renal compensatory mechanisms then bring about excretion of extra H^+ and returns the buffer system to normal. But in uncompensated **metabolic acidosis,** H^+ ion remain high.

Similarily in **metabolic alkalosis,** plasma HCO_3^- level and pH rise. **Respiratory compensation:** Decrease in ventilation produced by decline in H^+ concentration and this elevates PCO_2. This brings pH back toward normal while elevating HCO_3^- level further.

Renal compensation: More renal H^+ secretion is expanded in reabsorbing the increased filtered load of HCO_3^- and if HCO_3^- level in plasma exceeds 26.28 meq/l, HCO_3^- starts appearing in urine.

The rise in PCO_2 inhibits renal compensation by facilitating acid secretion but its effect is relatively slight.

9. In a patient with a plasma pH of 7.10, the [HCO_3^-] [H_2 CO_3] ratio in plasma is:

A. 20
B. 10
C. 2
D. 1
E. 0.1

Ans. (B)

Explanation:

[HCO_3^-] ratio	20	0.9	10	16
[H_2CO_3] pH	7.4	6.0	7.1	7.3

(Pg. 733)

10. In a patient who has become dehydrated, body water should be replaced by intravenous infusion of:

A. Distilled water
B. 0.9% sodium chloride solution
C. 5% glucose solution
D. Hyperoncotic albumin
E. 10% glucose solution

Ans. (C)

[illegible]

Similarly in metabolic alkalosis, plasma HCO_3^- [illegible]. Respiratory compensation: Decrease in ventilation [illegible] H^+ concentration [illegible] HCO_3^- [illegible]

Renal compensation: [illegible] renal H^+ secretion [illegible] HCO_3^- [illegible]

9. In a patient with a plasma pH of 7.1, the HCO_3^-/H_2CO_3 ratio in plasma is:

A. [illegible]

B. [illegible]

C. [illegible]

D. [illegible]

Ans. [illegible]

Explanation:

[illegible]

10. In a patient who has [illegible] contraindicated?

A. [illegible]

B. [illegible] solution

C. [illegible]

D. Hyperventilation

E. [illegible] solution

Ans. [illegible]